THE BIOCHEMISTRY OF

EXERCISE AND

METABOLIC ADAPTATION

THE BIOCHEMISTRY OF EXERCISE AND METABOLIC ADAPTATION

WAYNE C. MILLER, Ph.D.
Department of Kinesiology
Indiana University
Bloomington, Indiana

 Brown &
Benchmark

Library of Congress Cataloging in Publication Data:

MILLER, WAYNE C., 1954

THE BIOCHEMISTRY OF EXERCISE AND METABOLIC ADAPTATION

Cover Design: Gary Schmitt

Copy Editor: Vickie West

Library of Congress Catalog Card Number: 91-77406
ISBN: 0-697-16707-0

Printed in the United States of America by Brown & Benchmark, 2460 Kerper Boulevard, Dubuque, IA 52001.

10 9 8 7 6 5 4

Contents

ACKNOWLEDGMENTS

A million thanks are expressed to my wife, Patrice, who patiently supported me as I progressed through the development of this book. I also thank my parents for a lifetime of nurturing that enabled me to become who I am.

I would also like to acknowledge the contributions from all of the scientists who continually strive to discover truth. In light of the fact that this is not a comprehensive text, I give a sincere apology to any of those scientists who think that I may have underemphasized or possibly overlooked their contribution to the understanding of the biochemistry of exercise and metabolic adaptation.

PREFACE

The purpose of this book is to provide the student with an understanding of the biochemical principles that govern metabolic adaptation to exercise in skeletal muscle. It is intended to be used as a basic text for a class in exercise biochemistry, muscle physiology, or intermediary metabolism. It can also be used as a supplemental text for any exercise physiology course, as most exercise physiology texts only cover the biochemistry of exercise superficially and rarely introduce the student to the biochemistry that underlies the physiological adaptations to exercise training.

This book was not written to be comprehensive. As a supplemental text, it is brief enough to be manageable by upper-level undergraduates. On the other hand, there is enough depth in the book to provide a solid framework upon which a graduate professor can build a complete course without much effort.

The text is organized into nine chapters. Chapter 1 helps the student understand the structure and function of skeletal muscle, which is necessary before he or she can explore the metabolic consequences of exercise on skeletal muscle. Chapter 2 brings the student through the biochemical pathways that provide the energy for muscle contraction. These pathways include fat and protein catabolism, which are rarely covered sufficiently in physiology texts. However, the chemistry is presented in a manner simple enough for the unexperienced student to understand and is a great review for the student with a biochemistry background. Chapter 3 illustrates how surplus energy is stored when energy demand from exercise is reduced. Chapter 4 explains how energy production for muscle contraction is regulated.

Chapters 5 through 9 deal with the adaptations that occur within skeletal muscle as a result of exercise training. First, Chapter 5 presents the ultrastructural changes that occur within muscle itself in response to training. Next, Chapter 6 discusses the metabolic adaptations to very intense training. Then Chapter 7 illustrates the muscle's response to anaerobic training, and Chapter 8 follows with the metabolic adaptations resulting from aerobic training. The final chapter (9) briefly discusses the changes in hormonal responses to exercise following training. This text promises to be enlightening as well as stimulating for the serious student of exercise science.

PRELUDE

Exercise physiology is a sub-discipline of physiology dealing with changes in body function brought about by participation in physical exercise. As physical exercise is the aftermath of chemical reactions that transform chemical energy into mechanical energy, the understanding of the biochemistry of exercise is an integral part of exercise physiology. Many students shy away from exercise biochemistry because they feel that biochemistry itself has so many complex details that the thought of integrating biochemistry with exercise physiology becomes unfathomable. Exercise biochemistry need not be looked upon with anxiety. To the newcomer, the most complicated feature of this science is the necessity of becoming familiar with many new terms and modes of thinking. Once students gain this familiarity, however, they will enjoy delving deeper into the mysteries of exercise biochemistry.

PEDAGOGICAL AIDS

In order to help the student gain a quicker access to the biochemical dialogue, a list of some common biochemical terms and concepts used in this book follows.

Allosteric enzyme—In allosteric enzymes, the binding of a substrate to one active site of the enzyme can affect the binding of substrates to other active sites in the same enzyme molecule. The activity of an allosteric enzyme can be altered by regulatory molecules that are bound to sites other than the catalytic sites.

ATP—adenosine triphosphate. A nucleotide consisting of an adenine, a ribose, and a triphosphate unit. ATP is an energy-rich molecule that plays a central role as a carrier of free energy in biological systems. ATP is commonly referred to as the "energy currency" of the body because all energy produced in the body can be converted into ATP equivalents.

Coenzyme—a substance that is required in order for an enzyme to function. Many vitamins in the diet are precursors for coenzymes.

Condensation—a reaction where molecules are joined with the simultaneous elimination of another smaller molecule. Many times a condensation reaction is followed by a hydrolysis as in the formation of citrate from the condensation of oxaloacetate and acetyl coenzyme A (CoA).

Oxaloacetate + Acetyl CoA + H_2O $\leftrightarrow$ Citrate + HS-CoA + H^+

Deamination—a reaction where the NH_2 radical from an amino acid is lost. Some examples of deamination reactions are the deamination of serine, threonine, and alanine to pyruvate. The deamination of alanine is an oxidative deamination.

$$Serine \rightarrow pyruvate + NH_4^+$$
$$Threonine \rightarrow pyruvate + NH_4^+$$
$$Alanine + NAD^+ + H_2O \rightarrow puruvate + NH_4^+ + NADH + H^+$$

Decarboxylation—a reaction where a substance loses a molecule of CO_2. For example, here is the oxidative decarboxylation of pyruvate to form acetyl coenzyme A (CoA):

$$Pyruvate + CoA + NAD^+ \rightarrow Acetyl CoA + CO_2 + NADH$$

Dehydration—a reaction where a molecule of water is eliminated. An example of a dehydration reaction occurs when phosphoenolpyruvate is formed by the dehydration of 2-phosphoglycerate.

$$2\text{-phosphoglycerate} \leftrightarrow Phosphoenolpyruvate + H_2O$$

Enzyme—a protein that catalyzes the rate of a chemical reaction without being consumed in the reaction itself. Rates of biological reactions in the body are regulated by enzymes. Activation of an enzyme will increase the rate of a chemical reaction, whereas inactivation of an enzyme will inhibit the reaction.

Glycosidic Bond—Sugars can be linked to each other by O-glycosidic bonds to form disaccharides and polysaccharides. An oxygen atom is the common link between a carbon of one sugar and the carbon of another. Glycogen, the storage form of sugars in the liver and muscle, is a branched chain polysaccharide consisting of glucose molecules linked together by glycosidic bonds.

Hydrolysis—a reaction in which water is one of the reactants. In the context of this book, hydrolysis is a chemical decomposition in which a substance is split into simpler compounds by the addition of and the taking up of the elements of water. For example,

$$ATP + H_2O \leftrightarrow ADP + Pi + energy$$

Isomer—one of two or more chemical substances that have the same molecular formula but different chemical and physical properties due to a different arrangement of the atoms in the molecule.

Kinase—an enzyme that regulates a phosphorylation-dephosphorylation reaction.

Metabolite—a product of a metabolic reaction.

Mole—the chemist's unit of measure. A mole is that amount of an element having a mass in grams numerically equal to its atomic weight.

For example, 1 mole oxygen = 15.9994 grams oxygen. More precisely, there are 6.023×10^{23} atoms in one mole of an element.

NADH, FADH$_2$, NADPH—In the biological system, free energy is derived from the oxidation of fuel molecules (fat, carbohydrate, protein). In aerobic metabolism, the ultimate electron acceptor is oxygen. However, electrons are not transferred directly from fuel molecules to oxygen. Instead, the electrons are transferred to special electron carriers (NADH, FADH$_2$, NADPH) that then transfer the high energy-potential electrons to oxygen. As a result, ATP is formed. The newly formed ATP provides the energy for muscular contraction.

Oxidation/Reduction—A molecule is oxidized when it loses electrons in a reaction, and it is reduced when it gains electrons in a reaction. In the example below, pyruvate is reduced by NADH to form lactate. In the reverse reaction, lactate is oxidized by NAD$^+$ when pyruvate is reformed.

$$\text{Pyruvate} + \text{NADH} + \text{H}^+ \leftrightarrow \text{Lactate} + \text{NAD}^+$$

P:O Ratio—the ratio of the number of ATP formed to the number of atoms of oxygen consumed during oxidative phosphorylation.

Phosphorylation—a chemical reaction that adds a phosphate moiety (PO_3^{2-}) to a molecule or compound. Many enzymes are activated through phosphorylation. The oxidative phosphorylation of ADP (adenosine diphosphate) produces ATP (adenosine triphosphate), which supplies energy for muscular contraction.

Rate-limiting enzyme—an enzyme in a cascade of reactions that regulates the critical step in the cascade. The rate of flux through the cascade of reactions is determined or limited by the activity of the rate-limiting enzyme.

Respiratory Control—Electrons do not flow from fuel molecules to electron carriers and then to oxygen unless ADP is simultaneously phosphorylated to ATP. The most important factor in determining the rate of oxidative phosphorylation is the level of ADP. The regulation of the rate of oxidative phosphorylation by the ADP level is called respiratory control.

Substrate—the reactant molecule in a chemical reaction that binds to the enzyme regulating that particular reaction.

Thioester Bond—a bond where an oxygen molecule has been substituted with another molecule, often sulfur. For example, the bonding of CoA in Succinyl CoA is through a thioester bond where oxygen has been replaced by sulfur (Figure P-1).

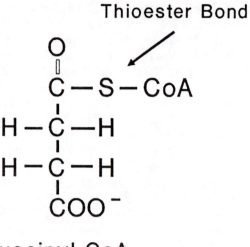

Figure P-1. Thioester bond in succinyl CoA.

Additional pedagogical aids can be found in the appendixes. Appendix A contains a list of common biochemical abbreviations used in this book. Appendix B provides the reader with a cross-reference among chapters and topics in this book and those of some of the most common exercise physiology textbooks on the market. This cross-reference will assist the student and professor who are using this book as a supplement to an exercise physiology text.

1

SKELETAL MUSCLE

The human body contains over 400 skeletal muscles which comprise about 45% of total body weight. Approximately 75% of skeletal muscle is water, 20% is protein, and the remaining 5% is made up of other substances such as fats, carbohydrates, high-energy phosphates, and minerals. Skeletal muscles are responsible for postural support as well as all body movement. A large portion of the metabolic activity of the body is for the purpose of sustaining muscular activity. During heavy exercise, the cellular metabolic rate can increase 50 times above the minimal resting requirement. Intermediary muscular metabolism is therefore the process of converting the chemical energy, originating from various food sources, into the mechanical energy necessary for body movement. A basic understanding of the structure and function of skeletal muscle is a prerequisite to the elucidation of the biochemical changes that occur during exercise.

THE STRUCTURE OF SKELETAL MUSCLE

Individual muscles are separated from each other and held in position by connective tissue called fascia (Figure 1-1). Just underneath the fascia, surrounding the whole muscle, is a layer of connective tissue called the epimysium. Moving inward from the epimysium, the muscle is divided into compartments that contain numerous muscle fibers (muscle cells). Groups of muscle fibers are enclosed by the perimysium. Each of these groups of muscle fibers is known as a fasciculus. Every muscle fiber within a fasciculus is surrounded by another layer of connective tissue called the endomysium. Thus, all parts of a skeletal muscle are enclosed in layers of connective tissue, that form a network extending throughout the entire muscle.

Individual muscles are made up of many parallel muscle fibers that usually run the entire length of the muscle. Almost all muscle fibers (98%) are innervated by only one nerve ending located near the

1

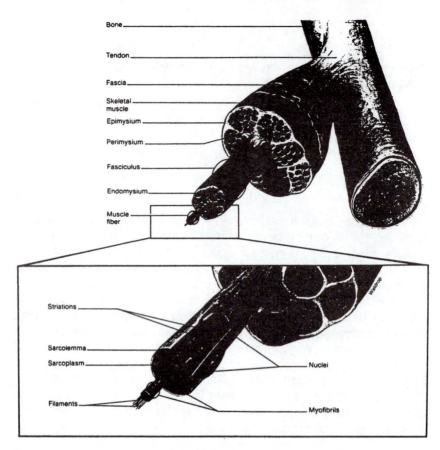

Figure 1-1. Anatomy of skeletal muscle and surrounding connective tissue. From: Hole, J.W. Jr., *Human Anatomy and Physiology*, 5th Ed. (1990). Dubuque, IA: Wm. C. Brown Publishers. Reprinted by permission.

middle of the fiber (Figure 1-2). Each fiber responds to nervous stimulation by contracting and then relaxing. Beneath the endomysium of a muscle fiber lies the sarcolemma, which is similar to the cell membrane of other types of cells. The sarcolemma encloses the sarcoplasm (cytoplasm). The sarcoplasm of the fiber contains the same organelles that are present in other cells. However, unlike other cells of the body, muscle fibers contain many nuclei. Another distinguishing characteristic of muscle fibers is their striated appearance (Figures 1-2 and 1-3). These striations are due to the unique arrangement or crossbanding of the myofibrils, which contain the protein filaments that are fundamental to the contraction mechanism.

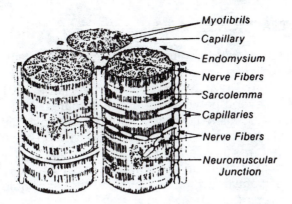

Figure 1-2. Nervous innervation of skeletal muscle fibers. From: Fox, E.L., et al., *The Physiological Basis of Physical Education and Athletics*, 4th Ed. (1988). W.B. Saunders Company. Reprinted by permission of Wm. C. Brown Publishers, Dubuque, IA.

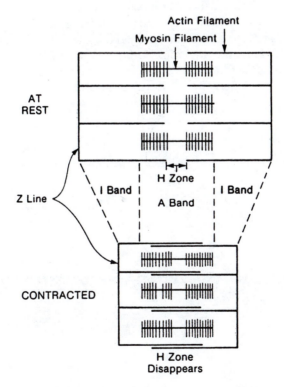

Figure 1-3. Skeletal muscle ultrastructure. From: Fox, E.L., et al., *The Physiological Basis of Physical Education and Athletics*, 4th Ed. (1988). W.B. Saunders Company. Reprinted by permission of Wm. C. Brown Publishers, Dubuque, IA.

THE CONTRACTION PROCESS

Within the myofibril are two protein filaments, one thick and one thin. The thick filament consists almost entirely of myosin protein molecules (Figure 1-4). The myosin molecule is very large (530 kilodaltons) and contains several polypeptide chains (Figure 1-4). Two identical heavy chains (230 kilodaltons) wrap around each other in a spiral to form a double helix or an α-helical coiled-coil rod (Figure 1-5). This portion of the myosin molecule provides a connecting link to similar units in the myosin filament. One end of each of these helical chains is folded into a globular protein mass called the myosin head (Figure 1-5). Light chains (20 kilodaltons) are also part of the myosin head (Figures 1-5 and 1-6). These light chains help control the function of the head during the process of muscle contraction. Differences in the light- and heavy-chain composition in the myosin head demarcate a muscle fiber's speed of contraction, strength of contraction, and energetics. Light chains 1 and 2 have also been subclassified into two types: 1s and 2s, or 1f and 2f. The 1s and 2s chains are heavily expressed in slow muscle, whereas the 1f and 2f chains dominate in fast-contracting muscle. (See the following section on Skeletal Muscle Fiber Types for further explanation of fast and slow muscle fiber types.) Also on the myosin head is an actin binding site and an ATPase (adenosinetriphosphatase). The actin binding site is where the interaction between the thick

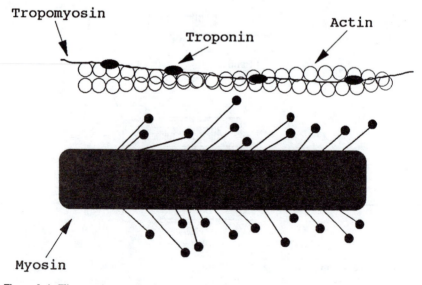

Figure 1-4. Filament interaction in muscle fibers.

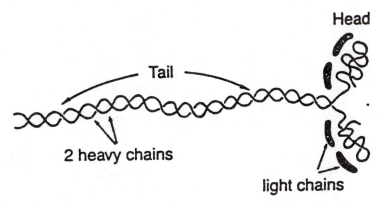

Figure 1-5. The myosin molecule. From: Guyton, A.C. (1991). *Textbook of Medical Physiology* (8th ed.). Philadelphia: W.B. Saunders, p. 70.

and thin filaments occurs during muscular contraction. ATPase is the enzyme that regulates the hydrolysis of adenosine triphosphate (ATP) to adenosine diphosphate (ADP) and inorganic phosphate (Pi). This hydrolysis of ATP ultimately provides the energy for muscular contraction.

$$\text{ATP} + H_2O \xrightarrow{\text{ATPase}} \text{ADP} + P_i + \text{energy}$$

The thin filament of the myofibril is also composed of several pro-

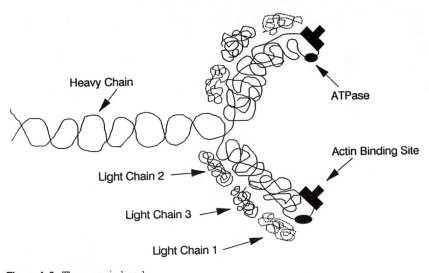

Figure 1-6. The myosin head.

teins. The primary protein that forms the backbone of the thin filament is actin. Actin can exist in two shapes, globular and fibrous. When the globular form (G-actin) polymerizes, it unfolds into the fibrous form (F-actin). The backbone of the actin filament is a helix of F-actin monomers. Attached to each one of the monomers of the helix is one molecule of ADP. It is believed that these ADP molecules are the active sites on the actin filaments that interact with the myosin filaments during muscle contraction.

Associated with the actin filament is another protein called tropomyosin (Figure 1-4). Molecules of tropomyosin, connected loosely with the F-actin strands, wrap themselves around the sides of the F-actin helix. At rest, the tropomyosin molecules inhibit interaction between actin and myosin by blocking the active sites on the actin strands.

Attached near one end of each tropomyosin molecule is yet another protein called troponin (Figure 1-4). The troponin is actually a complex of three protein subunits: troponin I, troponin T, and troponin C. Troponin I has a strong affinity for actin, troponin T a strong affinity for tropomyosin, and troponin C an affinity for calcium ions. The coordinated interaction of these protein subunits is what controls muscular contraction.

The actin filaments are attached to a Z membrane or Z line and extend on either side of the Z line (Figure 1-3). The Z line passes from myofibril to myofibril, attaching the myofibrils to each other all across the muscle fiber. The basic contractile unit of the muscle fiber is the sarcomere which extends from Z line to Z line (Figure 1-3).

In 1954, A.F. Huxley and R. Niedergerke in Cambridge, England, and H.E. Huxley and J. Hanson in Cambridge, Massachusetts proposed the *sliding filament theory* for muscular contraction. This theory states that the tropomyosin and troponin proteins regulate an interaction between the myosin and actin proteins of the thick and thin filaments. During the process of muscle contraction, cross-bridges attach between actin and myosin; the two filaments slide over each other when energy is provided by the hydrolysis of ATP to ADP and P_i.

$$ATP + H_2O \leftrightarrow ADP + P_i + energy$$

A skeletal muscle fiber normally does not contract until it is stimulated by a motor neuron. Each motor neuron normally branches several times and stimulates a few to several hundred skeletal muscle fibers. A motor neuron and all of the muscle fibers that it innervates constitute a motor unit. The site where the motor neuron and muscle fiber meet is called the neuromuscular junction (Figure 1-7). At this junction, the sarcolemma of the muscle fiber forms a pocket called the motor end plate. The process of muscular contraction begins with the

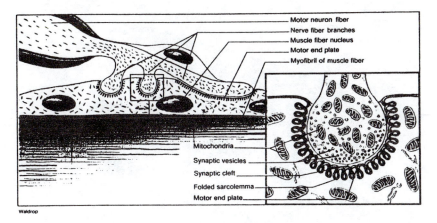

Motor neuron fiber
Nerve fiber branches
Muscle fiber nucleus
Motor end plate
Myofibril of muscle fiber

Mitochondria
Synaptic vesicles
Synaptic cleft
Folded sarcolemma
Motor end plate

Waldrop

Figure 1-7. The neuromuscular junction. From: Hole, J.W. Jr., *Human Anatomy and Physiology*, 5th Ed. (1990). Dubuque, IA: Wm. C. Brown Publishers. Reprinted by permission.

initiation of an action potential by the motor neuron and the transmission of the action potential across the motor end plate to the muscle fiber.

When a nerve impulse reaches the neuromuscular junction, about 200 to 300 vesicles of acetylcholine, a neurotransmitter, are released into the gap between the neuron and the motor end plate (Figure 1-7). The acetylcholine diffuses quickly across the gap and reacts with receptor molecules in the sarcolemma. This interaction between acetylcholine and receptor increases the permeability of the sarcolemma to sodium ions, resulting in the depolarization of the sarcolemma or an end-plate potential. If the end-plate potential is large enough to exceed threshold, the nerve impulse will be successfully transformed into a muscle impulse. As this muscle impulse is generated, it travels in all directions over the muscle fiber membrane while being transmitted deep into the fiber through a system of transverse tubules (Figure 1-8). The sarcoplasmic reticulum contains a high concentration of calcium ions, mostly stored in its cisternae (Figure 1-8). As the muscle impulse is transmitted throughout the fiber, the membranes of the cisternae become more permeable to calcium ions and the stored ions diffuse into the sarcoplasm of the muscle fiber.

In the absence of free calcium, the troponin of the thin filament inhibits interaction between the cross-bridges of the myosin and the actin molecule. Once free calcium is released into the sarcoplasm, it binds to the troponin. This calcium binding causes a positional change in the troponin molecule that also affects the positioning of the tropomyosin molecule. The result of the changing position of the troponin/tropomyosin complex is that the active sites for interaction between

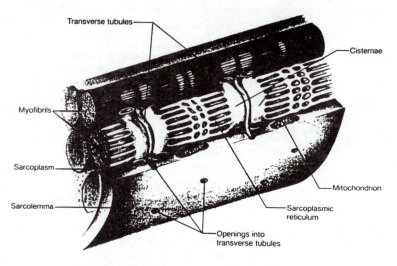

Figure 1-8. Communication network within the muscle sarcoplasm. From: Hole, J.W. Jr., *Essentials of Human Anatomy and Physiology*, 3rd Ed. (1989). Dubuque, IA: Wm. C. Brown Publishers. Reprinted by permission.

actin and myosin are now exposed on the actin molecule. This exposure allows for the contraction process to proceed (Figure 1-9).

ATP binds to the head of the myosin cross-bridge before contraction begins. The ATPase activity of the myosin head immediately hydrolyzes the ATP. Although the products of the reaction (ADP and P_i) remain bound to the myosin head, the head is now "energized" with the energy released during the reaction. The myosin head now interacts with the exposed binding sites on the actin filament. The binding of actin and myosin discharges the stored energy in the myosin head, altering the position of the myosin head and producing force through cross-bridge movement. As all of this occurs, the ADP and P_i previously attached to the head of the cross-bridge are released. A new molecule of ATP now binds to the site of release of ADP, causing detachment of the myosin head from the actin. After the myosin head is detached from the actin, a new molecule of ATP is hydrolyzed by the myosin ATPase. The hydrolysis of ATP energizes the myosin head again and the cycle can repeat itself for a new power stroke. Thus, the energy released from the hydrolysis of ATP is used to swivel the myosin cross-bridge in such a way that the thin filament (actin) slides over the thick filament (myosin). Since the myosin cross-bridges at each end of a sarcomere are oriented in opposite directions, the actin molecules which are attached to opposite Z lines of the sarcomere slide across the myosin towards each other, closing the H zone and shortening the length of the sarcomere (Figure 1-3).

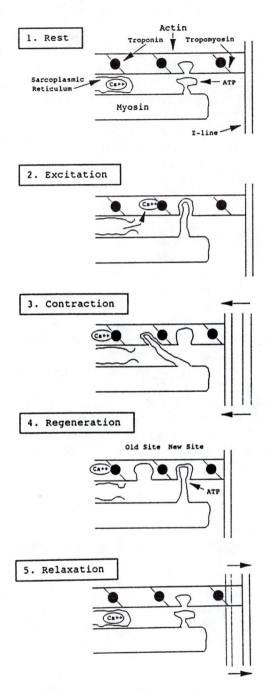

Figure 1-9. Sliding filament theory of muscle contraction.

Because a single contraction cycle of the myosin cross-bridges in a muscle can shorten the muscle by only 1% of its resting length, the contraction cycle must be repeated over and over for any significant shortening of the whole muscle. Attachment of a new ATP to a myosin cross-bridge allows the cross-bridge to detach from the actin and return to its original conformation. Once this occurs, the myosin can interact at a new position on the actin molecule.

Meanwhile, the acetylcholine that stimulated the contraction in the first place is rapidly being decomposed by the action of an enzyme called cholinesterase. Cholinesterase is present at the neuromuscular junction within the membranes of the motor end plate. The rapid removal of acetylcholine from the neuromuscular junction by cholinesterase insures that a single nerve impulse will not cause continued stimulation of a muscle fiber. The usual duration of an impulse in skeletal muscle is about 20 milliseconds. In order for muscle contraction to continue, there must be continual nervous stimulation of the muscle fiber. The signal to stop contraction, then, is the absence of the nerve impulse at the neuromuscular junction. When nervous stimulation of the muscle fiber stops, a continually active calcium pump located in the walls of the longitudinal tubules of the sarcoplasmic reticulum pumps calcium ions out of the sarcoplasm back into the cavities of the sarcoplasmic reticulum and its cisternae. The action of the calcium pump decreases the calcium concentration in the sarcoplasm, and this in turn removes the calcium from the troponin molecule of the thin filament of the myofibril. As calcium dissociates from the troponin, the troponin/tropomyosin complex returns to its original conformation and the active sites on the actin molecule are again inhibited from interacting with the myosin cross-bridges. The fiber has returned to its relaxed position.

The energy released from splitting a phosphate bond on the ATP molecule is critical to muscular contraction. Furthermore, a continuous supply of ATP is necessary to sustain muscular activity during exercise. Many of the biochemical adaptations that occur with exercise training are in response to the high demand for ATP-supplied energy. Future chapters of this book will reveal how the energy demand of exercise is met by the synthesis and hydrolysis of ATP through the metabolism of fat, carbohydrate, and protein.

The following dialogue is a summary of the events that occur during skeletal muscle contraction (see Figure 1-9).

1. **REST**   (a) Actin and myosin uncoupled
                     (b) Calcium stored in sarcoplasmic reticulum
2. **EXCITATION**   (a) Nerve impulse generated

                   (b) Acetylcholine released from vesicles
                   (c) Sarcolemma depolarized
                   (d) Muscle impulse transmitted through fiber
                   (e) Calcium released from cisternae
                   (f) Calcium binds to troponin
                   (g) Actin binding sites activated
                   (h) Myosin ATPase activated

3. **CONTRACTION** (a) $ATP \rightarrow ADP + P_i + energy$
                   (b) Myosin cross-bridges swivel
                   (c) Actin slides over myosin

4. **REGENERATION** (a) ATP resynthesized
                   (b) ATP attaches to myosin
                   (c) Actin and myosin dissociate
                   (d) Contraction process repeats

5. **RELAXATION** (a) Acetylcholine decomposed
                   (b) Nerve impulse stops
                   (c) Calcium removed by calcium pump
                   (d) Actin binding sites inhibited
                   (e) Muscle returns to resting state

The previous discussion reveals how muscle contraction is regulated by the concentration of calcium ions surrounding the filaments of the myofibril. Release of calcium is initiated by communication of the action potential from the sarcolemma via the transverse tubules to the sarcoplasmic reticulum. Although the mechanism of this communication is unknown, there are several theories proposed. Each of these theories carries some support as well as opposition. Although further research is needed before these theories receive universal acceptance, they warrant some reflection.

The postulate behind the calcium-induced calcium release hypothesis is that the stimulation of the transverse tubules induces a release of calcium from the transverse tubule membranes, perhaps from the cytoplasmic surface (Fabiato, 1985; Frank, 1982). This release of calcium from the tubule membranes in turn triggers the opening of calcium channel gates within the sarcoplasmic reticulum. Arguments against this hypothesis are based on problems with the amount of calcium required to induce release (Endo, 1977) and on the fact that blocking the calcium release channels on the cell membrane does not inhibit calcium release from the sarcoplasmic reticulum nor reduce tension development (McCleskey, 1985).

Another theory is that the voltage-induced changes in the transverse tubules induce the formation of D-myo-inositol 1,4,5-triphosphate (IP_3). IP_3 subsequently increases the permeability of the sarcoplasmic reticulum membranes to elicit calcium release (Nosek et al., 1986;

Vegara, Tsien, & Delay, 1985; Volpe et al., 1985). Support for this hypothesis comes from experiments demonstrating elevated production of IP_3 in skeletal muscle following electrical stimulation, the release of calcium in skinned muscle fibers induced by IP_3, an augmented skeletal muscle response following inhibition of IP_3 breakdown, and a reduction of calcium transients in skeletal muscle following repression of IP_3 release from red blood cells (Vegara, Tsien, & Delay, 1985). However, it has been questioned whether the concentration of IP_3 required for activation and its rate of activation are physiological (Walker et al., 1987).

It also has been suggested that activation of calcium release is due to perturbation of the normal H^+ gradient across the sarcoplasmic reticulum membranes (Dugan & Martinosi, 1970). However, the pH changes during muscle contraction may be too small to induce the necessary gradients in order to stimulate calcium release (Baylor, Chandler, & Marshall, 1982; Martinosi, 1984).

SKELETAL MUSCLE FIBER TYPES

Although the contraction process for all skeletal muscle is the same, not all muscle fibers have the same biochemical or functional characteristics. Skeletal muscle fibers are generally classified according to their primary dependence on different metabolic pathways for the production of ATP. As we will discuss in forthcoming chapters, the ATP necessary for muscle contraction can be produced through either aerobic (oxygen utilizing) or anaerobic (non-oxygen utilizing) pathways.

Currently, much controversy exists over the use of the terms aerobic and anaerobic to describe the different energy-producing pathways. Traditionally, any pathway that lead to the complete oxidation of a substrate was considered aerobic, because oxygen was used as the final hydrogen acceptor in the metabolic pathway. In contrast, any pathway that did not utilize oxygen to completely oxidize a substrate was considered anaerobic. Lactate or lactic acid, which is produced when carbohydrates are not completely oxidized, has been the traditional marker of anaerobic metabolism. Early scientists assumed that the production of lactate during exercise was simply a reflection of the anaerobic state of the working muscle. However, several reasons are now known for lactate formation; no oxygen or insufficient oxygen supply is only one of them. Using traditional terminology, anaerobic pathways for producing ATP are much quicker than aerobic ATP production, but are limited by the amount of available substrates. In contrast, aerobic ATP production is slow, but not limited by substrate availability. More descriptive terms such as "rapid" (for anaerobic) and "slow" (for aerobic) may come into use in the future (Brooks & Fahey, 1984, p. 74). However, until there is a consensus in the literature, the terms anaerobic and aerobic will be used in this book to designate the rapid energy-producing pathways and the slow energy-producing pathways, respectively.

The muscle fibers recruited to contract quickly and for only short periods of time are anaerobic in nature. On the other hand, although the aerobic fibers are slower to contract, they are not as easily fatigued as the anaerobic fibers. Even though muscle fibers may be better suited for either anaerobic or aerobic work, they all have some capacity for both types of metabolism. Most muscles in the body have an even mixture of both fiber types. The percentage of respective fiber types contained in a given muscle is genetically determined and neuro-muscularly controlled.

The scientific literature shows considerable confusion about the best method for determining fiber types and about their proper nomenclature. A debate of these issues is beyond the scope of this text, but a brief discussion of the most common classifying procedure follows.

The most common method for determining fiber types is the myosin ATPase pH lability method. This histochemical procedure involves staining individual muscle cells from a small piece (20 to 40 mg) of muscle tissue for the presence of the enzyme myosin ATPase, the enzyme that regulates the hydrolysis of ATP to provide the energy for muscular contraction. Fibers with a high anaerobic capacity have large quantities of myosin ATPase when compared to aerobic fibers. The stability of the myosin ATPase enzyme in different fiber types is dependent upon pH. Therefore, when the pH of the incubation solution for a muscle sample is manipulated, the amount of stable enzyme that is stained will be fiber-type dependent. Other glycolytic (anaerobic) and oxidative (aerobic) enzyme profiles are also used for fiber typing as well as electron microscopy.

The aerobic-type fibers are also called type I or slow-twitch fibers. Briefly, these fibers have a high capacity for oxidative metabolism, a slow speed of contraction, and are slow to fatigue. The anaerobic fibers are called type II or fast-twitch and are usually subdivided into two categories. Type IIa fibers are sometimes considered intermediate in that they have a fast contraction speed and are highly developed for both aerobic and anaerobic metabolism. Type IIb fibers posess the greatest potential for anaerobic work, are fast contracting, and are easily fatigued. A type IIc fiber has been identified, but it is an undifferentiated fiber that may be involved in reinnervation or motor unit transformation. The type IIc fiber is also rare, and its functional significance has not been determined. We will limit our discussion to the type I, IIa, and IIb fibers. Table 1-1 lists some common terminology for each of these respective fiber types along with an example of a muscle that is most representative of that particular fiber type.

You can see from Table 1-1 that the nomenclature for the different fiber types is very much descriptive of the fiber characteristics. Table 1-2 describes in more detail most of the characteristics of the different fiber types.

Although no sex or age differences occur in fiber type distribution in muscle, variation among individuals, as well as variation among muscles of the same individual, may be large. Generally 45 to 55% of the muscle fibers are slow-twitch. However, athletes who are very successful in endurance activities usually demonstrate a predominance of slow-twitch fibers in the muscles specific to their sport. On the other hand, athletes who are very successful in sports requiring power and strength tend to have more fast-twitch fibers. Although evidence from a number of sources suggests elite endurance athletes often exhibit a high percentage of slow-twitch fibers, other studies have shown that knowledge of a person's predominant fiber type is of limited value in predicting the outcome of athletic performance (Campbell et al., 1979; Komi & Karlsson, 1978). The implications muscle fiber types have upon exercise performance will be discussed later.

REFERENCES

Baylor, S.M., Chandler, W.K., & Marshall, M.W. (1982). Optical measurements of intracellular pH and magnesium in frog muscle fibers. *J. Physiol. (London),* 331: 139-177.

Brooks, G.A. & Fahey, T.D. (1984). *Exercise physiology human bioenergetics and its applications.* John Wiley, New York. 3. Campbell, C.J., Bonen, A., Kirby, R.L., & Belcastro, A.N. (1979). Muscle fiber composition and performance capacities of women. *Med. Sci. Sports Exerc.,* 11: 260-265.

Campbell, C.J., Bonen, A., Kirby, R.L., & Belcastro, A.N. (1979). Muscle fiber composition and performance capacities of women. *Med. Sci. Sports Exerc.,* 11: 260-265.

Duggan, P.F. & Martinosi, A. (1970). Sarcoplasmic reticulum. IX. The permeability of sarcoplasmic reticulum membranes. *J. Gen. Physiol.,* 56: 147-167.

Endo, M. (1977). Calcium release from the sarcoplasmic reticulum. *Physiol. Rev.,* 57: 71-108.

Fabiato, A. (1985). Calcium-induced release of Ca^{2+} from the cardiac sarcoplasmic reticulum. *Am. J. Physiol.,* 245: C1-C14.

Frank, G.B. (1982). Roles of intracellular and trigger calcium ions in excitation-contraction coupling in skeletal muscle. *Can. J. Physiol. Pharmacol.,* 60: 427-439.

Komi, P.V. & Karlsson, J. (1978). Skeletal muscle fibre types, enzyme activities and physical performance in young males and females. *Acta Physiol. Scand.,* 103: 210-218.

Martinosi, A.N. (1984). Mechanisms of calcium release from sarcoplasmic reticulum of skeletal muscle. *Physiol. Rev.,* 64: 1240-1320.

McCleskey, E.W. (1985). Calcium channels and intracellular calcium release are pharmacologically different in frog muscle. *J. Physiol. (London),* 361: 231-249.

Nosek, T.M., Williams, M.F., Zeigler, S.T., & Godt, R.E. (1986). Inositol triphosphate enhances calcium release in skinned cardiac and skeletal muscle. *Am. J. Physiol.,* 250: C807-C811.

Vegara, J., Tsien, R.Y., & Delay, M. (1985). Inositol 1,4,5-triphosphate: A possible chemical link in the excitation-contraction coupling in muscle. *PNAS (USA)*, 83: 6352-6356.

Volpe, P., Salviati, G., Di Virgilio, F., & Pozzan, T. (1985). Inositol 1,4,5-triphosphate induces calcium release from sarcoplasmic reticulum of skeletal muscle. *Nature*, 316: 347-349.

Walker, J.A., Somlyo, A.V., Goldman, Y.E., Somlyo, A.P., & Trentham, D.R. (1987). Kinetics of smooth and skeletal muscle by laser photolysis of caged inositol 1,4,5 triphosphate. *Nature*, 327: 249-252.

Table 1-1. Skeletal muscle fiber type nomenclature.

Type I	Type IIa	Type IIb
Slow-twitch (ST)	Fast-twitch (FT)	Fast-twitch (FT)
Slow Oxidative (SO)	Fast Oxidative-Glycolytic (FOG)	Fast Glycolytic (FG)
ST Oxidative (STO)	FT Oxidative (FTO)	FT Glycolytic (FTG)
Red	Red	White
ST Red (STR)	FT Red (FTR)	FT White (FTW)
Aerobic	Intermediate	Anaerobic
Tonic	Phasic	Phasic
Representative Muscle:		
Soleus (S)	Red Vastus Lateralis (RV)	White Vastus Lateralis (WV)

Table 1-2. Skeletal muscle fiber type characteristics.

Characteristic	STR	FTR	FTW
Motor neuron size	small	large	large
Recruitment threshold	low	high	high
Motor neuron conduction velocity	slow	fast	fast
Contraction time	slow	fast	fast
Relaxation time	slow	fast	fast
Force production	low	high	high
Resistance to fatigue	high	low	low
Elasticity	low	high	high
Fiber diameter	small	large	large
Z Line thickness	wide	medium	narrow
Hypertrophic response to training	small	large	large
Predominant energy system	aerobic	aerobic/anaerobic	anaerobic
Mitochondrial density	high	high	low
Capillary density	high	medium	low
Myoglobin content	high	medium	low
Myosin ATPase activity	low	high	high
Anaerobic enzyme activity	low	high	high
Aerobic enzyme activity	high	high	low
Phosphocreatine stores	low	high	high
Glycogen stores	low	high	high
Triglyceride stores	high	medium	low

2

ENERGY FOR MUSCULAR CONTRACTION

Metabolism is defined as all of the physical and chemical changes that take place within an organism including growth, physical transformations, and chemical transformations. Metabolism involves two fundamental processes: anabolism or the building-up process, and catabolism or the breaking-down process. In Chapter 1 we briefly discussed how the catabolism or breakdown of ATP provided energy for muscular contraction. We will soon learn that ATP can be synthesized (anabolism) by the breakdown (catabolism) of foods. Obviously, ATP plays a critical role in these metabolic processes.

ADENOSINE TRIPHOSPHATE AND ATP EQUIVALENTS

ATP is involved not only in muscular contraction, but in almost every extended metabolic process. The adenylates (ATP, ADP, AMP) play an almost universal role in metabolism. For this reason, ATP is sometimes called the "energy currency" of the body. In other words, all energy can be transformed or converted into ATP equivalents. An ATP equivalent is the energy differential in the conversion of ATP to ADP and vice versa. This means that any given metabolite can be evaluated in terms of either ATP equivalents released during its catabolism or ATP equivalents required for its anabolism. Dietary carbohydrate, fat, and protein can now be evaluated in terms of ATP equivalents gained during their degradation, which is no different than expressing their energy value as calories released during their degradation. The advantage of expressing energy values as ATP equivalents is that it defines energy in the currency units actually used within the cell, which emphasizes the primary importance of ATP in the metabolic processes of the cell.

PHOSPHOCREATINE—ATP ENERGY SYSTEM

Because the power of a muscle fiber depends upon the rate that ATP can be supplied to drive contraction as well as upon the fiber's contractile properties, muscles have the capacity to convert ADP and Pi back to ATP in a short time so contraction can continue. Carbohydrate, fat, and protein supply energy for the regeneration of ATP, but the most immediately available energy source for anabolism of ATP is phosphocreatine. Phosphocreatine (PC) has a high-energy phosphate group similar to ATP. PC can easily donate a phosphate group to ADP to form ATP. This reaction is catalyzed by the enzyme creatine phosphokinase (CPK).

$$(CPK)$$
$$\text{Phosphocreatine} + \text{ADP} \rightarrow \text{Creatine} + \text{ATP}$$

PC is only used for the purpose of phosphorylating ATP. During the initial stages of intense exercise, PC can keep the concentration of ATP high so that muscular contraction can continue. Creatine will then be reversibly phosphorylated to PC at rest when the muscular demand for ATP-derived energy has been reduced. The reverse reaction is also catalyzed by CPK and uses ATP as the phosphate donor.

$$(CPK)$$
$$\text{ATP} + \text{Creatine} \rightarrow \text{Phosphocreatine} + \text{ADP}$$

Is this a paradox? How can ATP donate its phosphate group and associated energy to regenerate PC if the ATP has already been catabolized for muscular contraction? The answer lies in the fact that dietary nutrients are used to regenerate ATP during recovery from exercise; this "new" ATP regenerates PC. Figure 2-1 demonstrates that ATP is recycled at the expense of either PC or dietary nutrients. PC, however, can be recycled at the expense of dietary nutrients. Therefore, the only expendables are the dietary nutrients. Such energy-containing nutrients are necessary to sustain metabolic processses.

A limiting factor in this model for energy production during intense exercise is PC stores. PC cannot be regenerated during intense exercise because ATP-derived energy is being used for muscular contraction. Intramuscular PC stores can only supply the energy requirements during maximal exercise for about 10 seconds.

A supplementary method to regenerate ATP when ATP and PC stores are depleted is through a reaction that joins two ADP molecules in order to generate one ATP. This reaction is controlled by the enzyme adenylate kinase (also called myokinase) and is illustrated below.

Adenylate Kinase

$$ADP + ADP \leftrightarrow ATP + AMP$$

We will discuss later how maximal exercise performance is affected by the ATP-PC energy system and how this system responds to exercise training. We will also learn how dietary nutrients can supply the energy requirements for prolonged exercise performance at submaximal workload intensities.

CARBOHYDRATE CATABOLISM

Glycolysis

The second most available method for producing ATP for muscle contraction is through the anaerobic breakdown of glucose. This catabolic pathway for the breakdown of glucose is called anaerobic glycolysis. Anaerobic glycolysis involves a series of 10 enzymatically

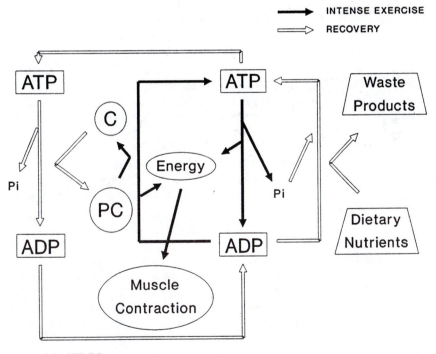

Figure 2-1. ATP-PC energy system.

controlled chemical reactions that break one glucose molecule down into two molecules of lactic acid or lactate. The glycolytic breakdown of glucose to lactate results in a net production of two ATP molecules. If the state of the muscle fiber favors complete oxidation of glucose, then the glycolytic pathway for glucose breakdown becomes aerobic glycolysis. Two molecules of pyruvic acid or pyruvate are formed during aerobic glycolysis rather than lactate as in anaerobic glycolysis. In short then, glycolysis results in the net production of two ATP and two molecules of either lactate or pyruvate for every glucose molecule catabolized.

As both anaerobic and aerobic glycolysis can occur simultaneously within the same cell or within the same muscle, there is overlap between anaerobic and aerobic metabolism. The metabolic fate of glucose entering the glycolytic pathway is not simply a matter of flipping a toggle switch between lactate and pyruvate formation. The ratio of lactate to pyruvate formation from glucose precursors depends upon several factors. These include enzyme kinetics, the mitochondrial capacity of the cell, hormonal control, oxygen availability, and the required rate of energy production. (See Brooks, 1985, 1988 for detailed review.)

Once glucose enters the muscle cell an irreversible phosphorylation reaction occurs. Phosphorylation of glucose effectively traps the glucose inside the sarcoplasm because phosphorylated sugars do not readily penetrate cell membranes. Glucose is now committed to further metabolism. The phosphorylation of glucose is catalyzed by the enzyme hexokinase (Figure 2-2). Hexokinase (HK) is one of the three regulatory enzymes of glycolysis. This first reaction in glycolysis is also rate-limiting. In other words, the rate of glucose flux through the glycolytic pathway is limited or controlled by the rate at which glucose is phosphorylated in the HK controlled reaction. HK is activated by high levels of glucose and inhibited by elevated levels of ATP and glucose 6-phosphate. One mole of ATP is expended for every mole of glucose phosphorylated. This means that energy is spent before any yield has occurred.

The second reaction in glycolysis is the isomerization of glucose 6-phosphate to fructose 6-phosphate. This reaction is catalyzed by phosphoglucose isomerase, is readily reversible, and is not rate-limiting. A second phosphorylation step follows the isomeration. Fructose 6-phosphate is phosphorylated by ATP to fructose 1,6-diphosphate. This phosphorylation also costs one mole of ATP per mole of glucose. Now there has been an investment of two ATP without any payback. The enzyme phosphofructokinase (PFK), which catalyzes this phosphorylation, is the most important rate-limiting enzyme in glycolysis. The activity of PFK is allosterically controlled by the concentrations of ATP

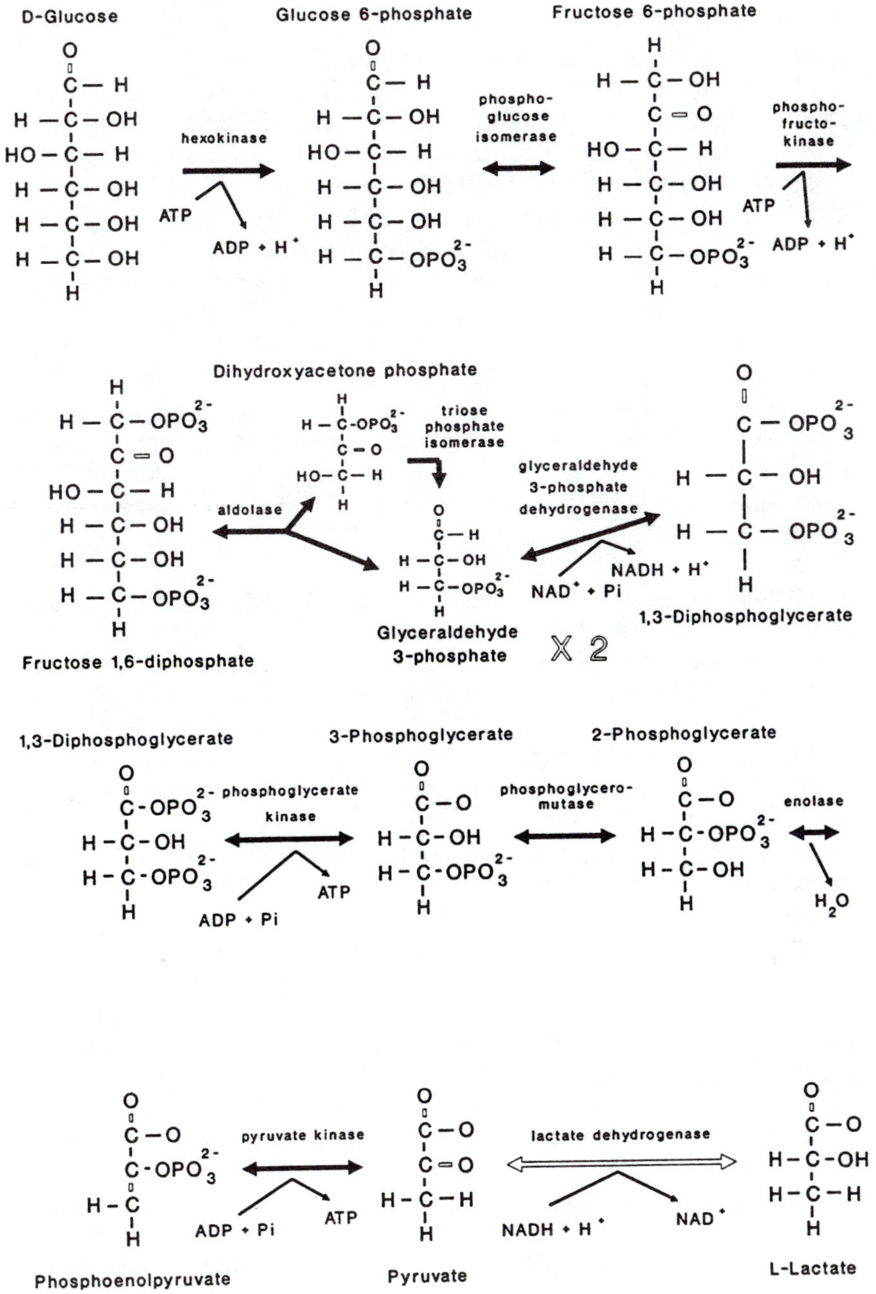

Figure 2-2. Glycolysis.

and fructose 6-phosphate as well as by other metabolites including fructose 2,6-diphosphate, citrate, ADP, and AMP.

Next, fructose 1,6-diphosphate is split into two 3-carbon units, dihydroxyacetone phosphate and glyceraldehyde 3-phosphate. This reaction is reversible and not subject to regulation. Dihydroxyacetone phosphate cannot proceed any further until it is isomerized into glyceraldehyde 3-phosphate by the enzyme triose phosphate isomerase. From this point on, everything is in duplicate because the 6-carbon glucose molecule has been converted into two 3-carbon glyceraldehyde 3-phosphate molecules.

The stage is now set for the production of ATP. Glyceraldehyde 3-phosphate will now be converted to 1,3-diphosphoglycerate in the first oxidation/reduction reaction of glycolysis. This reaction is regulated by glyceraldehyde 3-phosphate dehydrogenase. NAD^+ (nicotinamide adenine dinucleotide) accepts hydrogen ions that are released from glyceraldehyde 3-phosphate during the reaction. NAD^+ is a major electron acceptor in the oxidation of fuel molecules. During this process, called oxidation/reduction, NAD^+ accepts a hydrogen ion and two electrons as it becomes reduced to NADH. The NADH formed in this reaction will be reoxidized back to NAD^+ either by the conversion of pyruvate to lactate (anaerobic glycolysis) or through oxidation in the respiratory chain (aerobic glycolysis). Phosphoglycerate kinase catalyzes the next reaction in which 1,3-diphosphoglycerate is dephosphorylated to 3-phosphoglycerate and ATP (Figure 2-2). Now we are at the break-even point because two moles of ATP have been produced for the two that were invested.

The phosphoryl group on 3-phosphoglycerate now shifts to the second carbon atom to form 2-phosphoglycerate. This is a freely reversible reaction catalyzed by phosphoglyceromutase. The energy within 2-phosphoglycerate is redistributed as the molecule is dehydrated to form phosphoenolpyruvate. Enolase is the enzyme in this reversible reaction. This high-energy phosphate bond can now be used for ATP production. Fructose 1,6-diphosphate, the product of the PFK reaction, activates the enzyme pyruvate kinase which in turn regulates the formation of pyruvate with a concomitant production of ATP. This reaction is the third regulatory point of glycolysis. The net ATP production through the pathway is now two.

If the oxidation of pyruvate is not favorable, as in heavy exercise, the glycolytic production of ATP can continue only if NAD^+ is recycled by oxidizing NADH to NAD^+. This can happen if pyruvate is reduced to lactate. Therefore, a high $NADH/NAD^+$ ratio will favor lactate production. If the lactate produced accumulates in the muscle, it will lead to fatigue. On the other hand, lactate can diffuse into the blood and be converted to glucose in the liver or can be oxidized by the heart or the oxidative fibers of either the working muscle or non-working muscles (Brooks, 1988). The fates of lactate will be discussed in more detail later.

Glycogenolysis

The storage form of carbohydrate in the body is glycogen. Glycogen makes up 1 to 2% of wet muscle weight (400 g total) and about 6 to 10% of wet liver weight (100 g total). Muscle glycogen is used to synthesize ATP during muscular contraction. Liver glycogen is used to maintain blood glucose levels during fasting or the early stages of starvation. Glycogen itself is a branched-chain polysaccharide consisting only of glucose molecules linked together by glycosidic bonds. The primary bond is a 1-4 carbon linkage. After every 8 to 10 glucosyl units there is a branch formed by a 1-6 carbon linkage (Figure 2-3). Degradation starts as glycogen phosphorylase cleaves the 1-4 glycosidic bonds between residues at the nonreducing ends of the glycogen chains (Figure 2-3). A glucose 1-phosphate molecule is released with each cleavage. Glucosyl units are released from the chain until four units remain on each chain before a branch point. Phosphorylase cannot degrade the chain any further. At this time the enzyme glucosyl 4:4 transferase removes the outer 3 of the 4 glucosyl units attached at a branch and transfers them to the end of another chain. In other words, a 1-4 bond is broken and another 1-4 bond is made. The single glucose residue remaining is released by amylo 1:6 glucosidase. Glycogen phosphorylase can now continue working on the extended chain. The glucose 1-phosphate molecules released are converted to glucose 6-phosphate by the enzyme phosphoglucomutase and can now enter glycolysis. The free glucose released also enters the glycolytic pathway.

A summary of the main events occurring in the glycolytic pathway is presented in Figure 2-4. Carbohydrates in the form of glucose enter the pathway, are phosphorylated at the cost of 2 ATP (glucose 6-phosphate, fructose 1,6 diphosphate), split into two 3-carbon units (glyceraldehyde 3-phosphate), pass through a substrate level phosphorylation (1,3 diphosphoglycerate), phosphorylate four ADP molecules, and are converted to lactate (anaerobic glycolysis) or acetyl coenzyme A (aerobic glycolysis).

Citric Acid Cycle

The pyruvate formed during glycolysis will now be converted into one of three intermediary metabolites (Figure 2-5). As already mentioned, lactate will be formed if the required rate of energy production is high and aerobic metabolism cannot proceed to an appreciable extent. The formation of lactate recycles NAD^+ so that anaerobic production of ATP can continue. Pyruvate will be converted into acetyl

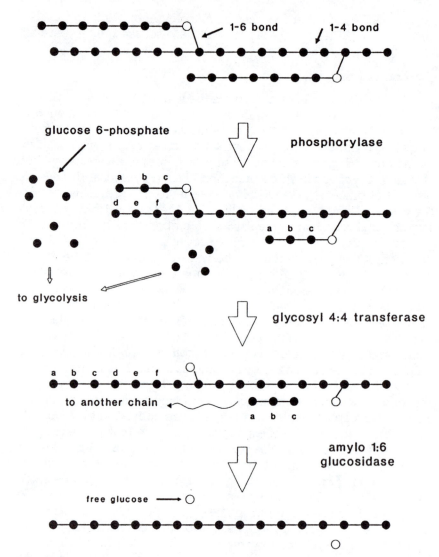

Figure 2-3. Glycogenolysis.

coenzyme A (CoA) when intracellular conditions favor aerobic catabolism of pyruvate. Acetyl CoA is the major fuel for the *citric acid cycle*, also known as the *Kreb's cycle* or *tricarboxylic acid cycle* (Figure 2-6). Pyruvate dehydrogenase is the enzyme that controls the conversion of pyruvate to acetyl CoA. This irreversible reaction is called oxidative decarboxylation and is important in muscle and the heart because of their high oxidative capacity. During the reaction, NAD^+ is reduced to NADH and carbon dioxide (CO_2) is released. The original glucose

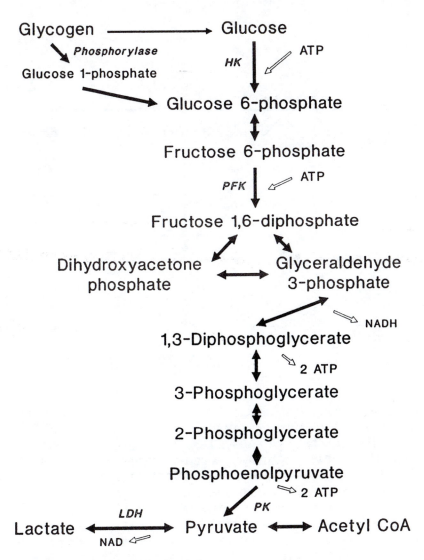

Figure 2-4. Summary of the main glycolytic events.

molecule has now been catabolized down to two 2-carbon (acetyl CoA) units.

The citric acid cycle (Figure 2-6) is the hub of all aerobic metabolism with acetyl CoA being a common metabolite for carbohydrate, fat, and protein catabolism. A 6-carbon unit called citrate is formed when oxaloacetate, which is a 4-carbon compound, condenses with the 2-carbon acetyl CoA and is subsequently hydrolyzed. This condensation/hydrolyzation is catalyzed by the enzyme citrate synthase. Citrate

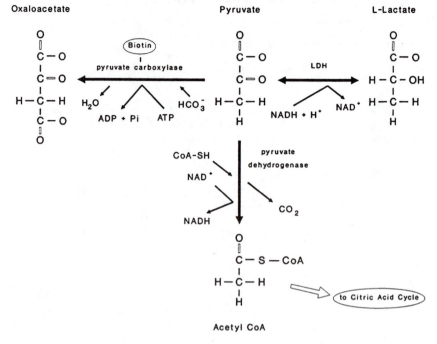

Figure 2-5. Metabolic fates of pyruvate.

synthase is an important regulator of the citric acid cycle and is inhibited by ATP, NADH, succinyl CoA, and acyl-CoA derivatives of fatty acids. The activity of citrate synthase is also affected by substrate availability. Next, citrate is isomerized to isocitrate in two reactions controlled by the enzyme aconitase. First, citrate is dehydrated to cis-aconitate, and then cis-aconitate is hydrated to form isocitrate. Isocitrate is now ready to undergo an oxidative decarboxylation reaction catalyzed by isocitrate dehydrogenase. CO_2 and the first of 3 NADH molecules produced by the cycle are released while α-ketoglutarate is formed. Isocitrate dehydrogenase activity is inhibited by ATP and NADH, which are both elevated when the muscle fiber has high energy stores. The second oxidative decarboxylation reaction occurs with the formation of succinyl CoA. Again CO_2 is released and the second NADH of the cycle is formed. (Notice that succinyl CoA is a 4-carbon intermediate.) The reaction is regulated by the α-ketoglutarate dehydrogenase enzyme complex. The energy from the thioester bond of succinyl CoA is used to phosphorylate GDP (guanosine diphosphate) into GTP (guanosine triphosphate) as succinate is formed. Because the energy content of ATP is the same as GTP, ATP is quickly formed in the following reaction:

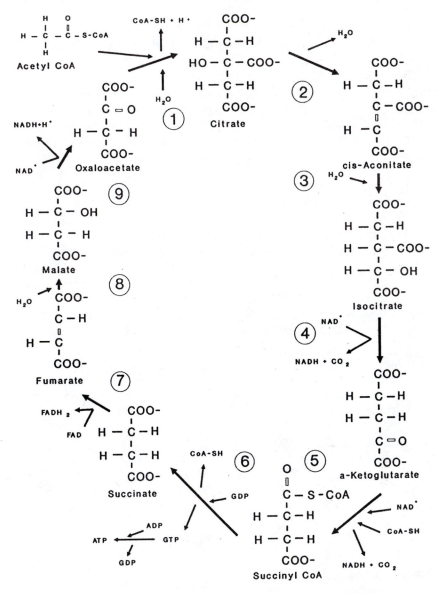

Figure 2-6. Citric acid cycle. Encircled numbers are symbolic for the following enzymes that govern the respective reactions. 1. Citrate synthase 2. Aconitase 3. Aconitase 4. Isocitrate dehydrogenase 5. α-Ketoglutarate dehydrogenase 6. Succinyl CoA synthetase 7. Succinate dehydrogenase 8. Fumarase 9. Malate dehydrogenase

Nucleotide Diphosphate Kinase

$$GTP + ADP \leftrightarrow GDP + ATP$$

Succinate is oxidized to fumurate in the succinate dehydrogenase controlled reaction, another key regulatory point in the citric acid cycle. FAD (flavin adenine dinucleotide) is reduced in this reaction rather than NAD^+. Fumarate is next hydrated to malate in a reversible reaction catalyzed by fumarase. Malate is subsequently oxidized to oxaloacetate in a reaction regulated by malate dehydrogenase. The third NADH molecule of the cycle is now formed and oxaloacetate has been regenerated. Remember that the cycle will turn two times for every glucose molecule catabolized.

Figure 2-7 summarizes the important events of the citric acid cycle with respect to the products produced and two key regulatory enzymes. A quick review of the cycle reveals that for every acetyl CoA molecule passing through the cycle 3 NADH are formed, 1 $FADH_2$, 1 ATP, and 2 CO_2. In other words, the products of the citric acid cycle are NADH, $FADH_2$, CO_2, and ATP. This does not seem a very efficient way of producing ATP when compared to anaerobic glycolysis as only 2 more ATP molecules have been generated per glucose molecule. However, a more abundant production of ATP comes when NADH and $FADH_2$ participate in the oxidative phosphorylation of ADP in the electron-transport chain. Before we proceed to the electron-transport chain, let us go back and discuss the third possible fate of pyruvate produced in glycolysis (Figure 2-5).

Pyruvate can also be carboxylated to oxaloacetate by the enzyme pyruvate carboxylase at the cost of an ATP. Pyruvate carboxylase contains biotin, which serves as a carrier of activated CO_2. The activity of pyruvate carboxylase depends upon the presence of acetyl CoA. A high level of acetyl CoA stimulates the enzyme by signaling the need for more oxaloacetate (Figure 2-6). This reaction is important because it replenishes citric acid cycle intermediates and also provides substrates for gluconeogenesis (formation of new glucose) from non-carbohydrate precursors.

Electron Transport Chain

The NADH and $FADH_2$ formed in glycolysis and the citric acid cycle are energy-rich molecules because they contain a pair of electrons that have a high-energy transfer potential. When these electrons are transferred to molecular oxygen, a large amount of energy is liberated which can be utilized to phosphorylate ADP. During the process, the electrons associated with the hydrogen atoms of NADH and $FADH_2$ are donated to a set of electron carriers collectively called the *electron transport chain* (Figure 2-8). The components of the electron transport

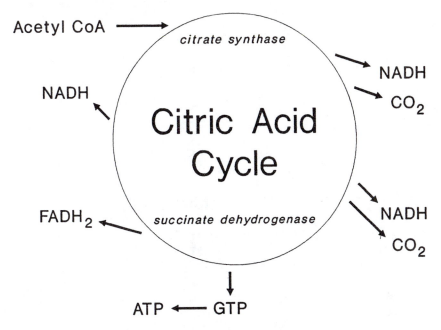

Figure 2-7. Summary of the main citric acid cycle events.

chain are located in the inner mitochondrial membrane. Electrons are transferred from one carrier in the chain to the next until they reach the end of the chain where they combine with oxygen and protons to form water. As the electrons are passed down the transport chain, they lose much of their free energy. Part of this energy is captured to produce ATP and part is lost as heat. The electron transport process accounts for most of the body's requirement for oxygen and is often referred to as the respiratory chain.

In the first step of the electron transport chain, two electrons are transferred from NADH to flavin mononucleotide (FMN) to form $FMNH_2$. FMN is part of a NADH dehydrogenase complex that is embedded in the inner mitochondrial membrane. Energy released during this transfer is used to phosphorylate ADP (ATP synthesis site #1). The electrons are next transferred to coenzyme Q (CoQ). CoQ can accept hydrogen atoms from both $FMNH_2$ and $FADH_2$. (The FMN moiety of the NADH dehydrogenase complex cannot accept hydrogens from $FADH_2$ because $FADH_2$ is at a lower energy state than NADH. Thus, $FADH_2$ enters the electron transport chain after the first site of ATP synthesis.)

The remaining members of the electron transport chain are cytochromes. Cytochromes are proteins containing a heme group that is different from that found in hemoglobin. Each cytochrome can carry only one electron rather than two as with NADH, $FMNH_2$, and CoQ.

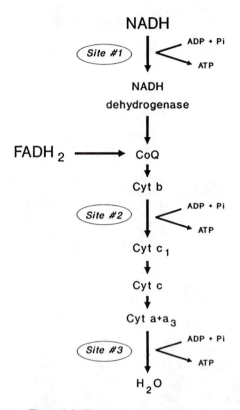

Figure 2-8. Electron transport chain.

Electrons are passed from CoQ to cytochromes b and c1 at which point a second ATP is formed (ATP synthesis site #2). The electrons continue to be transferred from cytochrome c_1 to cytochromes c, a, and a_3. Cytochromes a and a_3 exist as a complex sometimes called cytochrome oxidase. Cytochrome a_3 finally transfers the electrons to molecular oxygen. The third molecule of ATP is synthesized at this time. Thus, for every NADH that enters the transport chain 3 ATP are formed, and for every $FADH_2$ entering, 2 ATP are formed. The difference in the standard reduction potential between members of the electron transport chain allows the transfer of electrons to continue throughout the chain. The change in free energy produced by the passage of a pair of electrons from one member to the next is sufficient to produce ATP at three different sites (Figure 2-8).

The question remains as to how the oxidation of NADH is actually coupled to the phosphorylation of ADP? The most widely accepted hypothesis for this coupling phenomenon is the chemiosmotic theory of oxidative phosphorylation proposed by Peter Mitchell. This theory states that electron transport and ATP synthesis are coupled by a proton gradient across the inner mitochondrial membrane. In this model, the transfer of electrons through the electron transport chain causes protons from the mitochondrial matrix to be pumped to the other side of the inner mitochondrial membrane (Figure 2-9). The high concentration of positively charged hydrogen ions in the outer chamber and the large electrical potential difference across the inner membrane cause the hydrogen ions to flow preferentially into the mito-

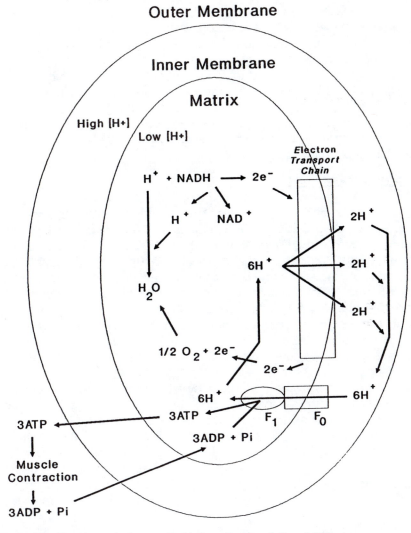

Figure 2-9. Chemiosmotic theory of oxidative phosphorylation of ADP.

chondrial matrix through the F_0-F_1 complex. The F_0 subunit is the proton channel of the complex, whereas the F_1 subunit is the coupling factor that contains ATP synthase. The hydrogen flow resulting from the pH gradient and membrane potential existing at the gate of the F_0-F_1 complex therefore constitutes a proton-motive force that is used to drive ATP synthesis.

Some NAD^+ is reduced to NADH in the cytosol during glycolysis. In order for NADH to be oxidized via the electron transport chain, it needs to traverse the inner mitochondrial membrane. Because the inner membrane is impermeable to NADH, the transfer of reducing equivalents from cytosolic NADH is accomplished via the malate-aspartate and/or glycero-phosphate shuttles. Using the glycero-phosphate shuttle, the reducing equivalents from cytosolic NADH are transferred to FAD with a corresponding drop in energy potential. On the other hand, in the malate-aspartate shuttle, the reducing equivalents from cytosolic NADH are transferred to NAD^+. Thus, when the glycero-phosphate shuttle is operative, the net production of ATP for each glucose molecule oxidized is 36; when the malate-aspartate shuttle is used, then the net ATP production is 38.

LIPID CATABOLISM

Fat is the other major nutrient that provides energy for muscular contraction. Approximately 95% of the fat in the body is in the form of triacylglycerols or triglycerides (TG). TG is simply a glycerol molecule attached to three fatty acids (Figure 2-10). Although most TG is stored in the fat cells, some is also found in the circulation and muscle cells themselves. TG is ideal for metabolic energy because it is highly reduced. Muscle fibers cannot oxidize TG directly but must first break it down to its glycerol and fatty acid components. The breakdown of a TG starts with the removal of a fatty acid from either the first or third glycerol carbon (Figure 2-10). This hydrolytic reaction is controlled by a TG lipase called hormone-sensitive lipase. Specific lipases for the remaining diacylglycerol and monoacylglycerol remove the remaining fatty acids. If the TG hydrolysis occurs in a fat cell, the glycerol and fatty acids will enter the circulation. Circulating glycerol will then be taken up by the liver and phosphorylated to glycerol 3-phosphate. Glycerol 3-phosphate can in turn be used to form more TG or can be converted to dihydroxyacetone phosphate, which can enter either the glycolytic or gluconeogenic pathways. The circulating free fatty acids will be taken up by the muscles where they can be further catabolized.

Once the fatty acid enters the muscle cell, it will be converted to a CoA derivative by the action of fatty acyl CoA synthetase (Figure 2-10). The fatty acyl CoA is now ready for β-oxidation, the major path-

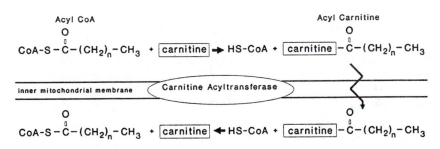

Figure 2-10. Triglyceride hydrolysis and fatty acid activation.

way for fat catabolism. β-oxidation is simply the successive removal of two-carbon fragments from the fatty acyl chain (Figure 2-11). These two-carbon fragments are actually acetyl CoA which can enter the citric acid cycle.

Since β-oxidation occurs in the mitochondria, the fatty acyl CoA first must be transported across the mitochondrial inner membrane. The transport process is called the carnitine shuttle because carnitine carries the acyl CoA through the inner mitochondrial membrane and then releases it in the motochondrial matrix (Figure 2-10). The enzyme that regulates this transport is carnitine acyltransferase. The fatty acyl CoA that is now in the mitochondrial matrix is free to enter the β-oxidation pathway.

The first reaction in β-oxidation (Figure 2-11) is the oxidation of fatty acyl CoA to enoyl CoA by fatty acyl CoA dehydrogenase. FAD is the hydrogen acceptor in this reaction. Next, enoyl CoA is hydrated to hydroxyacyl CoA by enoyl CoA hydratase. A dehydration step follows that produces ketoacyl CoA and NADH. Hydroxyacyl CoA dehydrogenase is the key enzyme in this reaction and also is a rate-limiting enzyme in the whole pathway. The final step is a thiolytic cleavage that releases a molecule of acetyl CoA. The acetyl CoA that is released can enter the citric acid cycle. The remaining fatty acyl CoA, now two car-

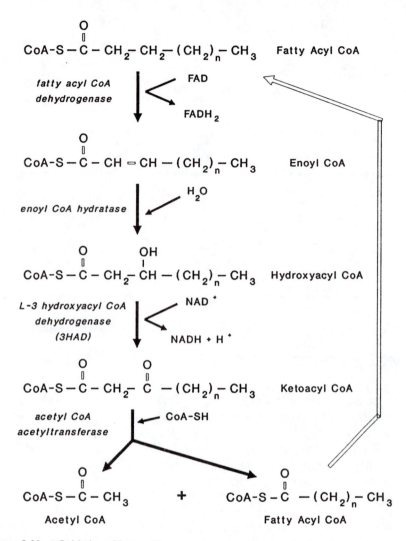

Figure 2-11. β-Oxidation of fatty acids.

bons shorter, repeats the cycle. The most common fatty acids oxidized contain 16 to 18 carbons. Palmitate, a 16-carbon fatty acid requiring 7 reaction cycles, yields a net of 129 ATP when oxidized.

The oxidation of a fatty acid with an uneven number of carbon atoms proceeds through the same steps as that of fatty acids with an even number of carbons until the final three carbons are left. This 3-carbon fatty acyl CoA is called propionyl CoA and is metabolized by converting it into succinyl CoA (Figure 2-12).

Acetyl CoA that is formed in the β-oxidation pathway enters the

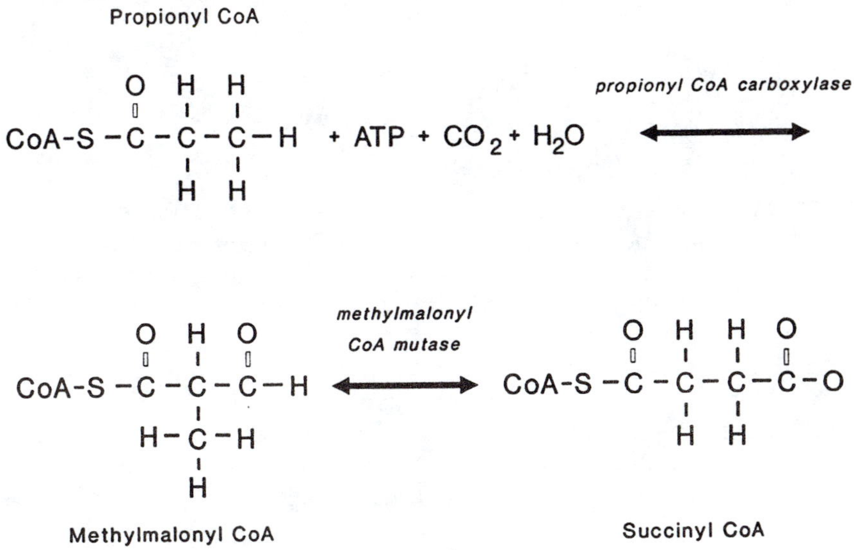

Propionyl CoA

$$\text{CoA-S} - \overset{\overset{\displaystyle O}{\|}}{C} - \overset{\overset{\displaystyle H}{|}}{\underset{\underset{\displaystyle H}{|}}{C}} - \overset{\overset{\displaystyle H}{|}}{\underset{\underset{\displaystyle H}{|}}{C}} - H \quad + \text{ATP} + CO_2 + H_2O \quad \xrightleftharpoons{\qquad} \quad$$ *propionyl CoA carboxylase*

methylmalonyl
CoA mutase

$$\text{CoA-S} - \overset{\overset{\displaystyle O}{\|}}{C} - \overset{\overset{\displaystyle H}{|}}{\underset{\underset{\underset{\displaystyle H}{|}}{\underset{\displaystyle H - C - H}{}}}{C}} - \overset{\overset{\displaystyle O}{\|}}{C} - H \quad \xrightleftharpoons{\qquad} \quad \text{CoA-S} - \overset{\overset{\displaystyle O}{\|}}{C} - \overset{\overset{\displaystyle H}{|}}{\underset{\underset{\displaystyle H}{|}}{C}} - \overset{\overset{\displaystyle H}{|}}{\underset{\underset{\displaystyle H}{|}}{C}} - \overset{\overset{\displaystyle O}{\|}}{C} - O$$

Methylmalonyl CoA   Succinyl CoA

Figure 2-12. Catabolism of propionyl CoA, a 3-carbon fatty acyl CoA.

citric acid cycle if an even balance between fat and carbohydrate degradation is present, or, in other words, enough oxaloacetate for the formation of citrate. When the breakdown of fat predominates and/or oxaloacetate availability is reduced, as in fasting, diabetes, and prolonged heavy exercise, acetyl CoA is diverted to the formation of ketones or ketone bodies. Two molecules of acetyl CoA will condense to form acetoacetate. Acetoacetate will be reduced to 3-hydroxybutyrate if the NADH:NAD+ ratio is high in the mitochondria. Otherwise, acetoacetate will undergo a slow spontaneous decarboxylation to acetone. The formation of these three ketones occurs primarily in the liver. The ketones formed in the liver diffuse into the blood and can be subsequently used for energy production, especially in the heart and kidney.

PROTEIN CATABOLISM

The principle constituents of proteins are the 20 amino acids that combine in unique arrangements to form each individual protein. All of the amino acids have two features in common, an amino radical (NH_2) and a carboxyl group (COOH). The remainder of the amino acid, which is called the side chain, can take on many forms and is composed of carbon, hydrogen, and sometimes sulfur or nitrogen. The specific structure of the side chain is what gives the amino acid its distinctive characteristics.

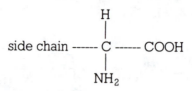

$$\text{side chain} \text{------} \overset{\overset{\displaystyle H}{|}}{\underset{\underset{\displaystyle NH_2}{|}}{C}} \text{------} COOH$$

Ten of the amino acids cannot be synthesized in the body and therefore must be supplied by the diet. These are called essential amino acids because they are essential to the diet. The remaining amino acids, called non-essential amino acids, can be synthesized by the cells in sufficient quantities to meet cellular needs. Dietary proteins that contain the essential amino acids in the amount and ratio analogous to the amino acids in the body tissues are complete proteins. In contrast, incomplete proteins either lack one or more of the essential amino acids, or the proper ratio of amino acids. Diets containing predominately incomplete protein can eventually lead to protein malnutrition.

When the amino acids from the diet enter the circulation, they become part of the body's amino acid pool. The three compartments of the amino acid pool are the blood, liver, and skeletal muscle. Amino acids in these compartments are in equilibrium, meaning amino acid metabolism in one compartment will affect the amino acids in the other compartments. Communication or exchange between the compartments is rendered by the blood. The benefit of this type of equilibrium among the compartments of the amino acid pool is that when dietary intake is temporarily insufficient, the metabolic needs of any one compartment can be met temporarily through relief from the other compartments. This benefit can be taken advantage of during very intense exercise or endurance exercise when energy stores in the muscle become depleted. Amino acids brought to the liver by the blood are converted into glucose (gluconeogenesis) and then released into the blood and delivered to the working muscles. This process is detailed and further explained by the *glucose-alanine cycle* (Figure 2-13).

In this model, amino acids in the muscle are converted into alanine and then released to the circulation. The liver takes the circulating alanine and removes the amino radical (deamination, Figure 2-14). The remaining carbon skeleton is converted into glucose and then released to the blood. The newly formed glucose is extracted from the blood by the working muscle and catabolized in order to support muscular contraction.

It has been estimated that after 4 hours of continuous exercise, the liver's output of alanine-derived glucose can account for 45% of the total glucose released from the liver (Ahlborg et al., 1974). In addition, as intensity of exercise increases, alanine release from exercising muscles

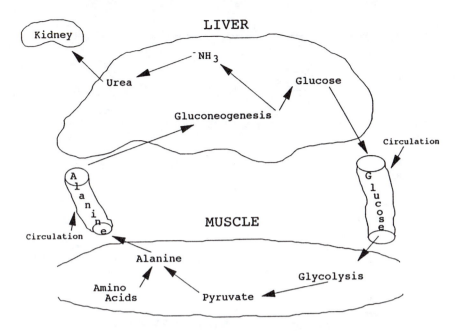

Figure 2-13. Glucose-alanine cycle.

increases by as much as sevenfold (Felig & Wahren, 1971). Energy derived from the glucose-alanine cycle may supply as much as 10 to 15%
of the total exercise requirement (McArdle, Katch, & Katch, 1991, p. 37).

Although protein is not a major source of energy during exercise,
amino acids in excess of those needed for synthesis of proteins must
be metabolized because they cannot be stored nor excreted. Amino
acid metabolism can be divided into two phases; disposal of the
α-amino group of the amino acid and catabolism of the remaining carbon skeleton. Urea is the disposal form of the α-amino groups derived
from amino acids. The process of urea formation is called the urea cycle (Figure 2-14). In this process, the α-amino group from the amino
acid is transferred to α-ketoglutarate to form glutamate, which is subsequently deaminated to yield ammonia (NH_4^+). The ammonia is then
converted into urea to be excreted. The carbon skeletons of the remaining α-ketoacid are then converted to common intermediates of intermediary metabolism (Figure 2-15). If the energy state of the cell is
high, amino acids can be converted to acetyl CoA and subsequently
stored as fat (see Chapter 3). If the energy state of the cell is low, amino
acids will be catabolized to support the energy demand of exercise. The
energy yield from each amino acid depends upon its entry point in the
citric acid cycle. Alanine, which enters via pyruvate, yields 15 ATP.

Figure 2-16 summarizes the main events in the different metabolic

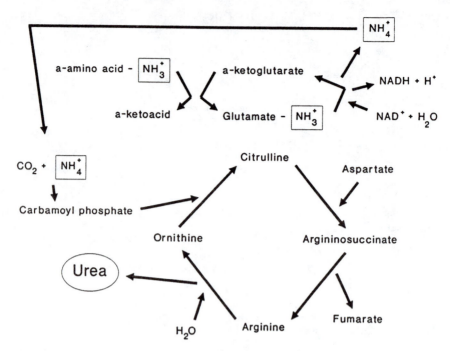

Figure 2-14. The urea cycle.

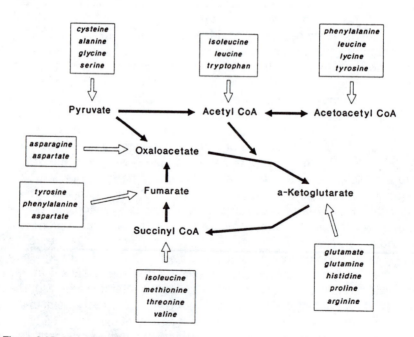

Figure 2-15. Metabolic fates of amino acids.

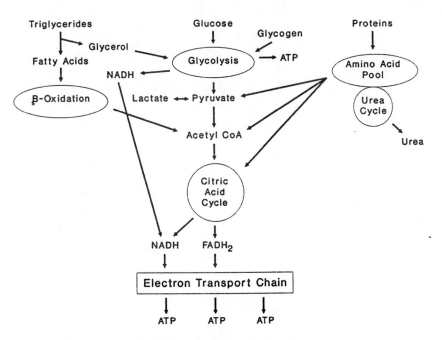

| Fat Catabolism | Carbohydrate Catabolism | Protein Catabolism |

Figure 2-16. Overview of interactions among catabolic pathways.

pathways for producing ATP from dietary nutrients. Although this diagram is not comprehensive, it helps one to piece together the different metabolic pathways in order to view intermediary metabolism as a whole. This figure may also serve as a quick reference for Chapters 4 through 9, where metabolic regulation and adaptation to exercise will be discussed.

REFERENCES

Ahlborg, G., Felig, P., Hagenfeldt, L., Hendler, R.,& Wahren, J. (1974). Substrate turnover during prolonged exercise in man. *J. Clin. Invest.*, 53: 1080-1090.

Brooks, G.A. (1985). Anaerobic threshold: Review of the concept and directions for future research. *Med. Sci. Sports Exerc.*, 17(1): 22-31.

Brooks, G.A. (1988). Blood lactic acid: Sports "bad boy" turns good. *Gatorade Sports Science Exchange*, 1(2): 1-4.

Felig, P. & Wahren J. (1971). Amino acid metabolism in exercising man. *J. Clin. Invest.*, 50: 2703-2714

McArdle, W.D., Katch, F.I., & Katch, V.L. (1991). *Exercise physiology energy, nutrition, and human performance.* (3rd ed.) Philadelphia, Lea & Febiger.

3

ENERGY STORAGE

If the energy supply to the body is in excess of that demanded for muscular contraction (and other physiological processes), then the surplus energy will be stored as either a carbohydrate or fat. Although diminished ATP and PC stores are replenished immediately after exercise stops (Figure 2.1), ATP and PC only account for a tiny amount of the energy stored in the body. Amino acids, which are not utilized for protein synthesis, cannot be stored as amino acids per se but must be converted to either a carbohydrate intermediate or fat. Glycogen is the primary storage form for carbohydrate whereas triglycerides (TG) are the primary storage form for fat.

GLYCOGEN STORAGE IN MUSCLE AND LIVER

In Chapter 2 we learned that glycogen is a branched chain polysaccharide consisting of glucose molecules linked together by a 1-4 or 1-6 glycosidic bond. Most of the body's glycogen is stored within the liver and muscles with a large variance in concentration between the two tissues as well as among the different muscle fiber types. Liver glycogen content responds primarily to dietary manipulation whereas muscle glycogen changes the most in response to exercise. Even though the liver has a higher concentration of glycogen (400 μmoles/g wet weight) than muscle (85 μmoles/g wet weight), the muscles contain the bulk of the body glycogen stores because of their larger mass.

Glycogen is made by adding one glucosyl unit at a time to an existing glycogen molecule and then rearranging the glycogen chains to make branches. The first step in the process of glycogen synthesis is the activation of glucose to make uridine diphosphate glucose (UDP-glucose), which subsequently becomes the glucose donor in the formation of glycogen. UDP-glucose is synthesized from glucose 1-phosphate and uridine triphosphate (UTP) in a reaction catalyzed by UDP-glucose pyrophosphorylase.

41

$$\text{Glucose 1-phosphate} + \text{UTP} + \text{H}_2\text{O} \leftrightarrow \text{UDP-glucose} + 2 \text{ Pi}$$

The UTP utilized in this reaction is generated by a nucleoside diphosphokinase reaction that uses ATP as the ultimate source of the high-energy phosphate.

$$\text{ATP} + \text{UDP} \leftrightarrow \text{ADP} + \text{UTP}$$

The second step in the synthesis of glycogen is the transfer of glucosyl units from UDP-glucose onto the residues in the growing glycogen chain. The activated glucosyl unit of UDP-glucose is transferred to the hydroxyl group at the C-4 terminal end of the glycogen chain and a 1-4 glycosidic bond is formed. This reaction is controlled by glycogen synthase, which is active only if a "primer" chain of 4 glucosyl residues is available.

The third step in glycogen synthesis is the formation of branches. Branching is necessary because it increases the solubility of the glycogen molecule. Theoretically, the glycogen synthase reaction could build a glycogen polysaccharide chain of indefinite length that consisted of only 1-4 bonds. However, the enzyme glycosyl 4:6-transferase takes a segment containing usually seven 1-4 residues from a chain of at least 11 residues and transfers it onto another chain at a point four residues from the nearest branch. During the transfer a 1-6 bond is formed. The new branch and the remaining branch from where it was taken can now grow in length by adding glucosyl units through the action of glycogen synthase.

It is not known for sure what limits the actual size of a glycogen molecule nor what limits the amount of glycogen stored within a tissue. Even under a heavy glucose load, excess glucose will be stored as fat. The overall storage efficiency of glycogen is rather high in spite of the cost of about 1 ATP per glucosyl unit. Most of the glucosyl residues of a glycogen chain will be phosphorolytically cleaved during glycogen degradation to glucose 1-phosphate which is converted at no cost into glucose 6-phosphate. The branch residues are hydrolytically cleaved and then phosphorylated into glucose 6-phosphate at the cost of one ATP. The net recovery of energy during glycogenolysis thus becomes about 97%.

GLUCONEOGENESIS

Prolonged exercise or fasting can deplete glycogen stores in addition to reducing blood glucose levels. In order to keep blood glucose levels constant when glycogen stores are compromised, a special pathway for glucose synthesis from non-carbohydrate precursors becomes active. The substrates for the formation of new glucose (gluconeo-genesis) are primarily lactate and α-ketoacids such as pyruvate, oxaloacetate, and α-ketoglutarate, all derived from metabolism of amino acids. Glycerol and any intermediate of glycolysis or the citric acid cycle can also give rise to the synthesis of glucose. Acetyl CoA and compounds that are converted to acetyl CoA cannot enter the gluconeogenic pathway because of the irreversible nature of pyruvate dehydrogenase, the enzyme that converts pyruvate to acetyl CoA. Thus, an important point to remember with respect to the physiology of energy storage, with particular significance to the development of obesity, is that *fat cannot be converted to carbohydrate, only catabolized or stored as body fat.*

The starting point of gluconeogenesis is pyruvate. Eight of the gluconeogenic reactions are simply reversals of glycolytic reactions. However, there are three glycolytic reactions that are irreversible (see Figures 2-4 and 3-1). These irreversible glycolytic reactions are bypassed by three new gluconeogenic reactions that favor glucose synthesis (Figure 3-1). The first barrier to overcome in the synthesis of glucose from pyruvate is the irreversible pyruvate kinase reaction. This barrier is bypassed by converting pyruvate to oxaloacetate in a carboxylation reaction catalyzed by pyruvate carboxylase. ATP is necessary in this reaction to drive the formation of the enzyme-biotin-CO_2 intermediate. Oxaloacetate is next decarboxylated and phosphorylated by PEP carboxykinase to make phosphoenolpyruvate. This reaction is driven by the hydrolysis of GTP.

The second barrier to overcome is the irreversible PFK reaction. This is bypassed with the hydrolysis of fructose 1,6-diphosphate by the enzyme fructose 1,6-diphosphatase. Another hydrolysis reaction overcomes the third barrier to glucose formation from pyruvate. Glucose 6-phosphatase is the gluconeogenic enzyme that bypasses the corresponding glycolytic enzyme hexokinase. Glucose formation in the gluconeogenic pathway is favored because of the irreversible formation of phosphoenolpyruvate, fructose 6-phosphate, and glucose; these latter are catalyzed by the gluconeogenic enzymes. The net cost of gluconeogenesis is six high-energy phosphate bonds.

FATTY ACID SYNTHESIS

The pathway for fatty acid synthesis is distinct from that of degradation. In fact, fatty acid synthesis occurs in the cytosol of the liver and adipose cells, whereas degradation occurs in the mitochondrial matrix. The overall synthetic process is an elongation of the growing fatty acid chain by sequential addition of two-carbon units derived from acetyl CoA (Figure 3-2). Fatty acid synthesis starts with the carboxylation of

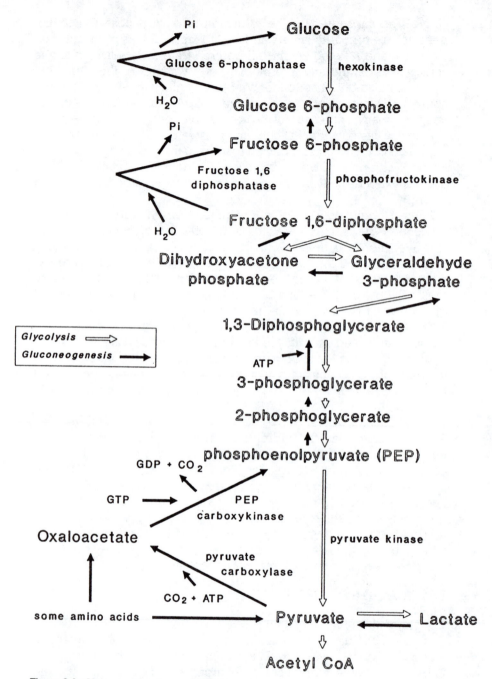

Figure 3-1. Gluconeogenesis vs. glycolysis.

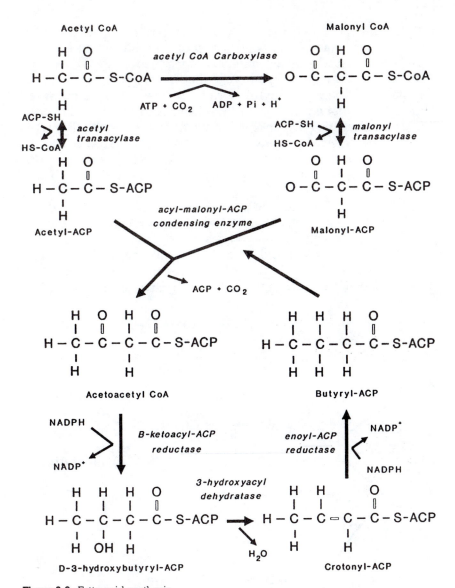

Figure 3-2. Fatty acid synthesis.

acetyl CoA to malonyl CoA. This irreversible step is regulated by acetyl CoA carboxylase which contains biotin as a CO_2 carrier similar to pyruvate carboxylase. The CO_2 donor is bicarbonate (HCO_3) whereas ATP provides the driving force. Next, another acetyl CoA and the newly formed malonyl CoA are linked to an acyl carrier protein (ACP). The enzymes, acetyl CoA transacylase and malonyl CoA transacylase, that catalyze these reactions are part of an enzyme complex called fatty acid synthetase. The condensation of acetyl-ACP and malonyl-ACP form acetoacetyl-ACP. This step is controlled by acetyl-malonyl-ACP condensing enzyme (part of the enzyme complex). A reduction step catalyzed by β-ketoacyl-ACP-reductase results in the formation of D-3-hydroxybutyryl-ACP. NADPH (nicotinamide adenine dinucleotide) is the reducing agent in contrast to NADH, as expected. Then D-3-hydroxybutyryl-ACP is dehydrated to form crotonyl-ACP. Finally, crotonyl-ACP is reduced to butyryl-ACP by NADPH. The butyryl-ACP can now condense with another acetyl-ACP to begin the elongation process again.

Fatty acids are synthesized in the cytosol, but acetyl CoA is formed from pyruvate in the mitochondria. Because acetyl CoA is not permeable to the mitochondrial membranes, citrate is formed to carry the acetyl CoA units across the mitochondrial membranes. Once the acetyl CoA is released in the cytosol, pyruvate is regenerated and can return to the mitochondria. This shuttle process is illustrated in Figure 3-3. No-

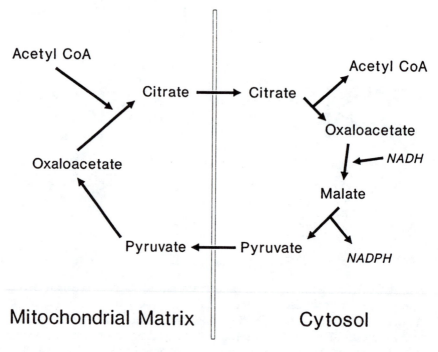

Figure 3-3. Transfer of acetyl CoA from the mitochondria to the cytosol via citrate.

tice how some of the NADPH needed for fatty acid synthesis is generated from cytosolic NADH. The remainder comes from the pentose phosphate pathway. In the pentose phosphate pathway, NADPH is generated when glucose 6-phosphate is oxidized to ribose 5-phosphate.

$$\text{Glucose 6-phosphate} + 2\,NADP^+ + 2H_2O \leftrightarrow$$
$$\text{Ribose 5-phosphate} + 2\,NADPH + 2\,H^+ + CO_2$$

The activity of the pentose phosphate pathway is very low in skeletal muscle, whereas it is very high in adipose tissue where large amounts of NADPH are utilized in the synthesis of fatty acids.

TRIGLYCERIDE SYNTHESIS

The synthesis of the TG molecule starts with the formation of glycerol 3-phosphate, the "backbone" upon which newly synthesized fatty acids can be attached. There are two pathways for glycerol 3-phosphate formation. In both the liver and adipose cells, glucose can be catabolized glycolytically to the point of dihydroxyacetone phosphate (DHAP). DHAP will then be reduced to glycerol 3-phosphate by glycerol 3-phosphate dehydrogenase. The second pathway exists in the liver only; glycerol is converted to glycerol 3-phosphate by glycerol kinase. The glycerol 3-phosphate from either source can now react with three fatty acids (fatty acyl CoA) to form the TG molecule.

The TG synthesis proceeds by the transfer of a fatty acid from its CoA derivative to the free hydroxyl group at position 1 of the glycerol 3-phosphate (Figure 3-4). The succeeding step is similar to the first and occurs at position 2. These two reactions are catalyzed by an acyl transferase. The resulting phosphatidate is hydrolyzed by a specific phosphatase that releases a phosphate and yields a diacylglycerol. This diacylglycerol is acylated in another transferase reaction resulting in the TG product.

TG that is synthesized in adipose tissue is stored in the cytoplasm. The TG remains stored in a highly concentrated form (anhydrous) until the demand for energy requires its mobilization. TG synthesized in the liver can combine with cholesterols, phospholipids, or proteins to form lipoproteins to be released into the circulation. Circulating TG molecules and their respective fatty acids are thus delivered to the peripheral tissues. More will be presented on the mobilization of fatty acids during exercise in Chapters 4 and 5.

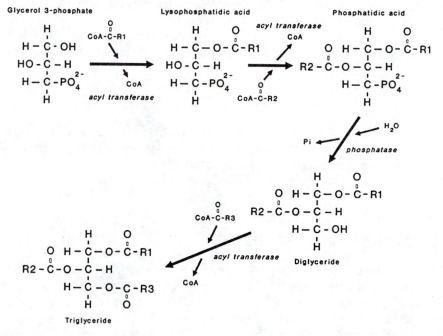

Figure 3-4. Triglyceride synthesis.

4

REGULATION OF ENERGY PRODUCTION DURING EXERCISE

WORK INTENSITY AND SUBSTRATE UTILIZATION

The primary sources for ATP in the exercising muscles are stored ATP, stored PC, anaerobic glycolysis, carbohydrate oxidation, and fat oxidation. Each of these sources can be evaluated in terms of either the total amount of ATP produced or its rate of ATP production. Table 4-1 contains the values reported for ATP production from each of these energy sources (Sahlin, 1985). Fat oxidation can produce the most amount of energy (moles ATP); however, the rate of energy production is very slow during fat oxidation. In contrast, immediate use of stored ATP can provide energy very quickly, but very little energy is available.

The relative intensity of exercise that can be supported by each energy source is also shown in Table 4-1. A clear relationship exists between maximal power output of an energy source and the relative exercise intensity that source can support. When the rate of ATP production is insufficient to meet the demand from exercise, the muscle becomes fatigued. Therefore, muscular fatigue and endurance must be expressed in the context of either exercise intensity or energy source. For example, very high intensity exercise can only be supported by the ATP and PC energy systems for about 32 seconds. The muscles will become fatigued at this time and exercise must cease unless the intensity is reduced. Anaerobic glycolysis cannot support *very* high intensity exercise, but will support high intensity exercise for about 7 minutes. Exercise for longer than 7 minutes will be supported by the oxidation of carbohydrates, but only at a lower intensity than anaerobic glycolysis. The energy reserve stored in fat can support exercise for several days, but the rate of ATP production is very low.

With this in mind, we generally talk about exercise endurance in terms of power endurance (ATP + PC systems), anaerobic endurance (glycolysis), and aerobic endurance (carbohydrate and fat oxidation).

49

Table 4-1. ATP production from the different energy sources.

Energy Source	Moles ATP Available	Max Power mmol ATP/kg dry muscle/sec	Relative Exercise Intensity Supported	Exercise Time
ATP stores	0.02	11.2	very high	1-2 sec
PC stores	0.34	8.6	very high	30 sec
Anaerobic Glycolysis	5.20	5.2	high	7 min
Carbohydrate Oxidation	70.00	2.7	moderate	90 min
Fat oxidation	8000.00	1.4	low	350 hr

Assuming a maximal oxygen consumption (max $\dot{V}O_2$) of 4.0 L/min, fat oxidation = 50% of max $\dot{V}O_2$, glycogen stores = 830 mmol (see Sahlin, 1985).

In other words, one level of fatigue is reached when ATP and PC stores become depleted. Another level of fatigue is reached when lactate levels rise and anaerobic glycolysis cannot continue. A third level of fatigue is reached when muscle and possibly liver glycogen become depleted. Depleted fat stores are not a limiting factor in exercise endurance.

In reality there is some overlap among the different energy sources or metabolic pathways. Energy required for exercise below 40 to 50% of $\dot{V}O_2$ max will be derived primarily from the oxidation of fat with some contribution from carbohydrate oxidation. As the intensity increases to around 50 to 70% of maximal aerobic capacity, additional oxidation of carbohydrate must occur because of the requirement for higher power output. At about 70% of $\dot{V}O_2$ max, the higher rate of energy production necessitates ATP production through anaerobic glycolysis. If the exercise intensity is further increased to near or above maximal aerobic capacity, the ATP and PC stores will be utilized for producing the energy necessary for muscular contraction.

A biochemical model of how exercise intensity determines which metabolic pathway will be utilized for ATP production during exercise has been presented by Hochachka and Somero (1984, pp. 113-124). In this model (Figure 4-1) the CPK enzyme exists in two isoforms. The cytosolic CPK phosphorylates ADP at the cost of PC as previously shown (Figure 2.1). The mitochondrial CPK rephosphorylates C and delivers ADP to the F1 ATP synthetases. This model proposes that during exercise the cytosolic CPK has a high affinity for ADP and can out-compete all other enzymes for the ADP liberated by the myosin ATPases. As cytosolic ADP concentration ([ ] = concentration) increases due to ATP being used for muscular contraction, [PC] also drops while [C] rises. This small change in cytosolic ADP concentration is thus transmitted to the F1 ATP synthetases in the mitochondria indirectly through increasing [C], which turns on the ADP shuttle. Once the shuttle is turned on,

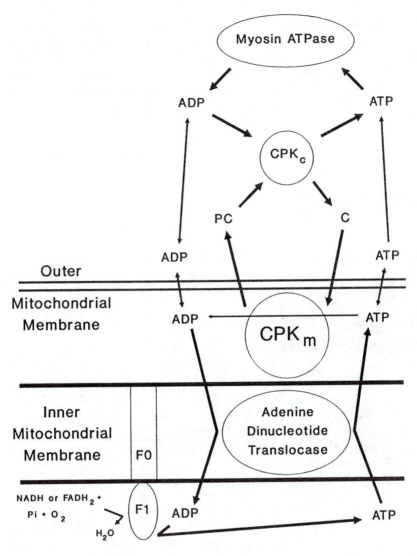

Figure 4-1. Biochemical model of how exercise intensity determines metabolic source for ATP production during exercise.

the F1 ATP synthetases will out-compete the cytosolic CPK for ADP. If enough oxygen is available to produce the ATP demanded by exercise (low intensity), oxidative phosphorylation will occur. If oxygen supply is limiting (very high intensity exercise), then cytosolic CPK will continue as the strongest competitor for the ADP, and PC stores will provide the necessary energy for muscular contraction.

Therefore, under conditions of very high intensity or low intensity exercise, small changes in [ADP] will activate the appropriate metabolic pathway, depending on oxygen availability and power output demand. Both of these conditions preclude any contribution from glycolysis. When the exercise intensity is too high for oxidative phosphorylation and the exercise duration is beyond that of the PC system, [PC] decreases with a concomitant increase in [ADP]. This elevation in [ADP] is greater than that seen during either low or very high intensity work. The significance is that large changes in [ADP] will activate the PFK and PK enzymes of glycolysis, whereas small changes in [ADP] will activate either the PC pathway or oxidative phosphorylation.

SPECIFIC REGULATORY POINTS
ALONG THE METABOLIC PATHWAYS

We have seen in Chapter 1 how the calcium-mediated events of the myofibrils regulate the activity of myosin ATPase and hence the contractile process. The preceeding discussion reveals how CPK responds to changes in [ADP] and [C]. Let's turn our attention now to some of the specific regulatory points along the glycolytic and oxidative pathways.

Phosphorylase Regulation

Glycogenolysis is controlled by phosphorylase as shown in Figure 2-3. The phosphorylase itself exists in two isoforms, phosphorylase b and phosphorylase a. Muscle phosphorylase b is active only in the presence of high levels of AMP (adenosine monophosphate). However, under most physiological conditions, phosphorylase b is inhibited by ATP and glucose 6-phosphate. Phosphorylase b can be converted to phosphorylase a, the more active isoform, simply by phosphorylating it. The sequence of events leading to the phosphorylation of phosphorylase b may seem complex at first, but it is a classic example of the principle of signal amplification in the biological system (Figure 4-2).

Glycogenolysis is activated primarily by two hormones, glucagon and epinephrine. Circulating levels of these hormones will interact with a specific receptor in the cell membrane of the liver or muscle cell. An enzyme called adenylate cyclase that is integrated within the cell membrane is stimulated by the hormone. Adenylate cyclase catalyzes the conversion of ATP to cyclic AMP. The newly formed cyclic AMP activates a protein kinase enzyme that serves two functions. Protein kinase activates a phosphorylase kinase while inhibiting the glycogen synthase enzyme. This coordinated regulation of glycogen synthesis and degradation is important so that ATP is not wasted in two opposing pathways. The activated phosphorylase kinase enzyme works upon phosphorylase b and converts it to the more active "a" form by a

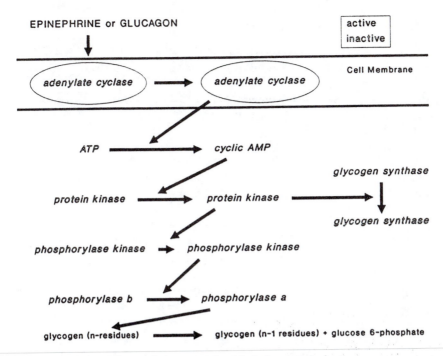

Figure 4-2. Epinephrine- and glucagon-stimulated glycogenolysis.

phosphorylation reaction. The phosphorylase a in turn stimulates glycogenolysis.

One might wonder why such a complicated series of events is necessary just to stimulate one enzyme. The purpose of the sequential steps is to amplify the hormonal signal. One epinephrine molecule received by a receptor will cause activation of several protein kinase molecules. Each of these will activate several phosphorylase kinase molecules which in turn activate many phosphorylase b molecules. The result is that many more glycogen molecules will be degraded by the enzyme cascade than if the hormone interacted only with the phosphorylase b.

Additional activation of glycogenolysis can occur without the phosphorylation of protein kinase. This happens when calcium from the sarcoplasmic reticulum of the muscle fiber is released into the sarcoplasm. The calcium binds to calmodulin, a calcium-binding protein that can activate enzyme systems when it binds calcium. The binding of calcium to the calmodulin subunit of the phosphorylase kinase activates phosphorylase b. This additional pathway for stimulation of glycogenolysis bypasses the phosphorylation of protein kinase.

Glycolytic Enzyme Regulation

The three regulatory enzymes in glycolysis are hexokinase (HK), phosphofructokinase (PFK), and pyruvate kinase (PK). HK is inhibited by high levels of glucose 6-phosphate and ATP. HK is activated, on the other hand, by elevated glucose levels. The PFK reaction is the rate-limiting step in glycolysis and is the most important control point. PFK is inhibited by high [ATP] and elevated amounts of citrate, which indicate plenty of energy within the cell. However, increased levels of AMP, ADP, fructose 2,6-diphosphate, and ammonia activate the enzyme. These activators are all metabolic byproducts that are elevated during exercise and help stimulate continued energy production through glycolysis.

PK is activated by fructose 1,6-diphosphate, the product of the PFK reaction. This type of feed-forward control of PK links the two kinase activities together. PK is inhibited by protein kinase. When blood glucose levels are low, protein kinase in the liver stimulates glycogenolysis. The inhibition of PK by protein kinase will shunt phosphoenolpyruvate from glycolysis toward gluconeogenesis to assist in elevating blood glucose.

Lactate dehydrogenase (LDH) is not in the glycolytic pathway per se, but it helps determine the fate of pyruvate during exercise. If cytosolic NADH production from glycolysis exceeds the oxidative capacity of the electron transport chain, the [NADH] will increase. This increase in [NADH] or the $NADH/NAD^+$ ratio favors the conversion of pyruvate to lactate by activating LDH. The end result is that glycolysis can continue because NAD^+ has been regenerated for the glyceraldehyde 3-phosphate dehydrogenase reaction (Figure 2-2).

Citric Acid Cycle Enzyme Regulation

Citrate synthase (CS) is a key regulatory enzyme in the citric acid cycle. The activity of CS is inhibited by elevated [ATP], [NADH], [acetyl CoA] and is activated by elevated [ADP]. CS activity is also controlled by intermediary substrates. If oxaloacetate levels drop dramatically, there will not be enough oxaloacetate to combine with acetyl CoA to form citrate. Hence, CS activity will be depressed. Additionally, citrate itself inhibits the CS enzyme. Working together then, an accumulation of citrate raises its concentration as an inhibitor while lowering the concentration of oxaloacetate as a substrate. The complete citric acid cycle must function at the same rate as the first step in order to restore the oxaloacetate consumed in the first step (Figure 2-6).

Another control point in the citric acid cycle is isocitrate dehydrogenase. This enzyme is stimulated by ADP; ADP enhances the enzyme-substrate affinity because of the mutually cooperative binding of isocitrate, NAD⁺, Mg²⁺, and ADP. On the other hand, isocitrate dehydrogenase is inhibited by ATP and NADH.

A third regulatory point in the citric acid cycle is α-ketoglutarate dehydrogenase. This enzyme is inhibited by succinyl CoA and NADH, the products of the reaction. In addition, a high energy charge in the cell will inhibit α-ketoglutarate dehydrogenase activity.

Although succinate dehydrogenase (SDH) is not usually considered a rate-limiting enzyme of the citric acid cycle, the fact that its activity responds to exercise training suggests an important regulatory role during exercise. SDH is inhibited by malonate, a dicarboxylic acid that differs from succinate in that it has one methylene group instead of two. SDH itself is not affected by substrate availability because whatever affects substrate supply to one enzyme of the cycle will affect all of the cycle.

Regulation of Cytochrome Oxidase in Electron Transport

The key enzyme in the regulation of electron flow through the electron transport chain is cytochrome a+a₃ or cytochrome oxidase (CO). CO is inhibited completely by cyanide. Cyanide poisoning is the same as oxygen deprivation because the final transfer of electrons to oxygen is blocked when CO is inhibited. CO responds to [ADP] as discussed previously. As mentioned earlier, the key to activation of the cytochrome enzymes is oxygen availability.

Enzymatic Regulation of Lipolysis

Triglyceride Lipases. The first step in the catabolism of TG is hydrolysis of the fatty acids from the glycerol backbone of the TG molecule. This step is catalyzed by the TG lipases. Hormone-sensitive lipase (HSL) is the specific TG lipase for the hydrolysis of adipose tissue TG. HSL is activated by cyclic AMP-dependent protein kinase, similar to when phosphorlylase b is converted to phosphorylase a in glycogenolysis. Epinephrine and glucagon are also the hormones that initiate the enzyme cascade resulting in HSL activation. On the other hand, high serum levels of glucose and insulin inhibit HSL.

Lipoprotein lipase (LPL) hydrolyzes circulating TG. Activity of this enzyme is also increased by cyclic AMP-dependent protein kinase (Oscai, Caruso, & Palmer, 1986) as well as by insulin (O'Looney, Maten, & Vahouny, 1983).

The intracellular TG lipase in muscle has not yet been positively identified. Evidence is mounting to suggest that HSL or an isoform of HSL, rather than a precursor for LPL, functions inside the muscle cell in the same way as adipose tissue HSL (Miller et al., 1989; Holm, Belfrage, & Fredrickson, 1987; Small, Garton, & Yeaman, 1989). Whichever enzyme regulates intracellular lipolysis in muscle, it is generally accepted to be under hormonal control through cyclic AMP. A link between lipid and carbohydrate metabolism exists because glycerol is readily interconvertible with the carbohydrate intermediates glycerol 3-phosphate and dihydroxyacetone phosphate. Thus, high levels of glucose oxidation shift the equilibrium between free fatty acids and triglycerides toward triglyceride storage, inhibiting fatty acid oxidation.

Carnitine Acyltransferase. The transport of acyl CoA derivatives across the mitochondrial membrane is catalyzed by carnitine acyltransferase (CAT). This enzyme is inhibited by malonyl CoA, a precursor for fatty acid synthesis. Therefore, when energy is abundant within the cell, surplus acetyl CoA will be diverted from the citric acid cycle to malonyl CoA, shutting down catabolism and opening up anabolism of fatty acids.

3-hydroxyacyl CoA Dehydrogenase. Although 3-hydroxyacyl CoA dehydrogenase is not necessarily rate limiting to β-oxidation, its activity will change in response to dietary manipulation and exercise as will be shown later. Its regulation is basically controlled through substrate availability.

HORMONAL CONTROL OF ENERGY PRODUCTION

Several hormones come into play as one exercises. Some of them affect the energetics of muscle contraction whereas others affect physiological processes related to exercise such as water balance, temperature regulation, and cardio-respiratory control. The hormones that affect the energetics of muscular contraction are glucagon, insulin, epinephrine, norepinephrine, and cortisol. A brief discussion of how these five hormones affect energy production during exercise follows. A more detailed review of the hormonal adaptations to exercise is presented in Chapter 9.

Glucagon

Glucagon is a hormone secreted by the alpha cells of the pancreas. Its function is to maintain blood glucose levels by stimulating glycogenolysis and gluconeogenesis in the liver. A reduction in blood glucose levels is the primary stimulus for glucagon secretion. However, epinephrine released either during exercise or in anticipation of exercise will stimulate glucagon release regardless of circulating levels of blood glucose. Glucagon exerts its influence in the cell through cyclic AMP-dependent protein kinase. Activated protein kinase stimulates glycogenolysis as shown in Figure 4-2. At the same time, protein kinase diverts carbohydrate intermediates from glycolysis to gluconeogenesis by inhibiting PFK and PK activities.

Insulin

Insulin is secreted by the beta cells of the pancreas and functions in direct opposition to glucagon. Insulin controls blood glucose metabolism of most tissues by regulating glucose transport into the cells. When blood glucose levels are elevated, insulin inhibits glycogenolysis and gluconeogenesis by counteracting the stimulation of adenylate cyclase seen with epinephrine and glucagon. TG synthesis is elevated in the fat cells when insulin provides more substrates for fatty acid synthesis by increasing the transport and metabolism of glucose in the cells. Insulin secretion is reduced when glucose levels drop and when epinephrine levels are elevated during exercise. Comparing the actions of insulin and glucagon to each other, one can consider insulin to be the "energy storage hormone" and glucagon to be the "energy use hormone".

Epinephrine and Norepinephrine

Epinephrine and norepinephrine are part of a group of biologically active amines called catecholamines. These two hormones are released from the adrenal glands in response to low blood glucose concentration and exercise or its anticipation. Most of the actions of these catecholamines are mediated through cyclic AMP. These actions include stimulation of glycogenolysis, lipolysis, and gluconeogenesis. In addition to the energetics of muscle contraction, the catecholamines affect cardiac output, respiration, blood pressure, and neuromuscular transmission during exercise.

Cortisol

Cortisol is the major glucocorticoid secreted by the adrenal cortex. It reduces glucose catabolism and stimulates glycogen synthesis. Cortisol promotes the breakdown of tissue proteins into amino acids that can be utilized by the liver for gluconeogenic reactions. Cortisol also stimulates gluconeogenesis by increasing synthesis of the amino acid deaminating enzymes. The gluconeogenetic effects of glucagon are supported by cortisol. The secretion of cortisol also depresses liver lipogenesis while accelerating the mobilization and use of fat for energy production during exercise.

REFERENCES

Hochachka, P.W. & Somero, G.N. (1984). *Biochemical Adaptation*, Princeton, NJ; Princeton University Press.

Holm, C., Belfrage, P., & Fredrickson, G. (1987). Immunological evidence for the presence of hormone-sensitive lipase in rat tissues other than adipose tissue, *Biochem. Biophys. Res. Comm.*, 148(1): 99-105.

Miller, W.C., Gorski, J., Oscai, L.B. & Palmer, W.K. (1989). Epinephrine activation of heparin-nonreleasable lipoprotein lipase in 3 skeletal muscle fiber types of the rat, *Biochem. Biophys. Res. Comm.*, 164(2): 615-619.

O'Looney, P., Maten, M.V., & Vahouny, G.A. (1983). Insulin-mediated modifications of myocardial lipoprotein lipase and lipoprotein metabolism, J. Biol. Chem., 258(21): 12994-13001.

Oscai, L.B., Caruso, R.A., & Palmer, W.K. (1986). Protein kinase activation of heparin-releasable lipoprotein lipase in rat heart, *Biochem. Biophys. Res. Comm.*, 135(1): 196-200.

Sahlin, K. (1985). Metabolic changes limiting muscle performance, In Saltin, B. (ed.), *Biochemistry of Exercise VI* (pp. 323-343). Champaign, IL; Human Kinetics.

Small, C.A., Garton, A.J. & Yeaman, S.J. (1989). The presence and role of hormone-sensitive lipase in heart muscle, *Biochem. J.* 258: 67-72.

5

MUSCLE ULTRASTRUCTURAL ADAPTATIONS TO EXERCISE TRAINING

One of the remarkable things about the human body is its tremendous ability to adapt to change. The driving force behind biological adaptation is a disruption in homeostasis. The remainder of this book will focus upon the adaptations that occur in muscle in response to the chronic disruption in energy homeostatis caused by exercise.

FIBER TYPE DISTRIBUTION IN EXERCISE-TRAINED vs. UNTRAINED MUSCLE

Muscle fiber type distribution is one of the first areas of interest relative to exercise-induced adaptation. Chapter 1 illustrates that skeletal muscle is composed of three primary fiber types, each of which is characterized by its functional capacity. A question often asked is how does the distribution of skeletal muscle fiber types affect exercise performance? Early investigations have revealed a direct relationship between fiber type distribution and specific exercise activity. For example, Gollnick et al. (1972) obtained muscle biopsy samples from the vastus lateralis and deltoid muscles of 74 trained and untrained men. Although a wide variety existed in fiber type distribution, slow-twitch (ST) fibers predominated in the muscles of the endurance athletes (aerobic training). By averaging values reported for the two untrained groups and the six endurance-trained groups in this study, percent distribution of ST fibers in the vastus lateralis was approximately 40% for the untrained and 60% for the endurance-trained. A similar difference was found for the deltoid muscle; 46% ST for the untrained and 60% for the endurance-trained (see Figures 5-1 and 5-2 for details). Edstrom and Ekbolm (1972) similarly studied fiber type distribution in weight lifters, endurance athletes, and untrained controls. Staining for myofibrillar ATPase distinguished the aerobic fibers (STR or slow-twitch red, and FTR or fast-twitch red) from the anaerobic fibers (FTW or fast-twitch white). Fifty-two percent of the vastus lateralis muscle fibers were aerobic in the endur-

VASTUS LATERALIS

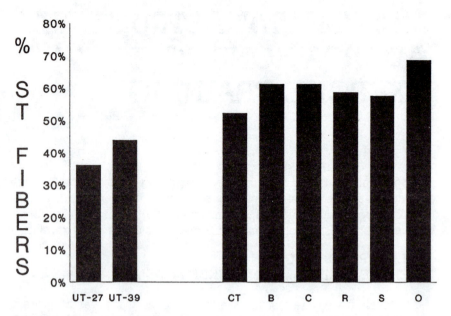

Figure 5-1. Fiber type distribution among athletes and nonathletes. UT-27 and UT-39 represent untrained groups with an average age of 27 and 39 years respectively. CT = Cross-trained. B = Bicyclists. C = Canoeists. R = Runners. S = Swimmers. O = Orienteers.

ance athletes, compared to 48% for the controls and only 44% for the lifters. These types of differences were also seen in a later study by Prince, Hikida, and Hagerman (1976) comparing vastus lateralis fiber type distributions among runners, power lifters, and sedentary subjects. Table 5-1 shows that the power lifters had a greater percentage of FTW fibers than the runners, and that the runners had a lower percentage when compared to controls. It is interesting to note that the FTR fibers comprised only a small portion of the vastus lateralis muscle in the power lifters. These data suggest that the primary difference in fiber distribution between aerobic and anaerobic athletes depends upon whether the FT fiber population in a muscle is of the anaerobic or aerobic type (FTW vs. FTR).

The distribution of FT fibers within the vastus lateralis muscle of endurance athletes, nonathletes, and elite weight lifters/power lifters was compared in a 1984 study by Tesch, Thorsson, and Kaiser. Endurance athletes had fewer FT fibers (40%) than both the nonathletes (60%) and the lifters (59%).

DELTOID

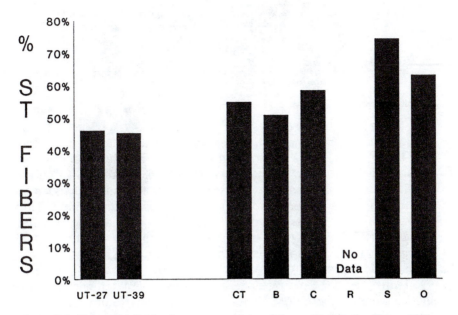

Figure 5-2. Fiber type distribution among athletes and nonathletes. See Figure 5.1 for abbreviations.

A difference in fiber type distribution between endurance-trained and nontrained muscles of the *same* athletes was found by Tesch and Karlsson (1985). Comparisons revealed that the percentage of ST fibers in the deltoid of kayakers was higher than in their vastus lateralis (71±11 vs. 41±10 %, p<0.001). On the other hand, the percentage of ST fibers in the deltoid of runners was lower than that of their vastus lateralis (49±8 vs. 67±10 %, p<0.01). The authors concluded that this pattern may reflect the adaptive response to long-term endurance training.

The data reviewed thus far are descriptive in nature in that they only describe differences between exercise-trained and untrained muscle. Such data may suggest that exercise training alters the composition of fiber types within a muscle but do not establish a cause and effect relationship.

Fiber Type Response to Aerobic Exercise Training

In order to determine whether the observed differences in fiber type distribution depend upon the effect of training or on genetic differences, Andersen and Henriksson (1977b) conducted a training study. Volunteer subjects (n=12) trained on a bicycle ergometer 30 minutes a

Table 5-1. Vastus lateralis fiber type distributions among power lifters, runners, and sedentary controls.

	% FTW	% FTR	% STR
Sedentary controls	26.2	38.1	35.5
Power lifters	33.3	10.5[+]	45.0
Runners	4.5[*]	39.7	44.3

[*]Significantly different from other groups, p<0.005.
[+]Significantly different from other groups, p<0.02.

day, 4 times a week, for 8 weeks at 81% of their $\dot{V}O_2$ max. Muscle biopsies were taken from the vastus lateralis before and after training. The data in Table 5-2 show a change in the expression of the FT fibers. The number of FTR fibers in the muscle increased 5% whereas the number of FTW fibers decreased 5%. Ingjer (1979) found similar changes in women who were subjected to 45 minutes of cross-country running for 24 weeks at 50 to 90% of $\dot{V}O_2$ max (Table 5-2). These data suggest that aerobic training promoted a transformation in the composition of the FT fibers in the exercised muscle without a change in the overall percentage of FT fibers.

More recently, Simoneau and associates (1985) demonstrated an increase in the number of STR fibers of the vastus lateralis muscle following high-intensity aerobic training. The proportion of the muscle taken up by the STR fibers was 41% prior to training and 47% after training. Consequently, the proportion of the muscle comprised of FTW fibers was reduced from 17% to 11%. The number of FTR fibers remained the same. Why changes were seen in the STR population during this training study and not during previous studies could possibly be due to the higher intensity and intermittant training protocol used by Simoneau's group.

An earlier study with guinea pigs also showed an exercise-induced increase in STR fibers with a corresponding decrease in FTW fibers and no change in the FTR fiber population (Barnard, Eggerton, & Peter,

Table 5-2. Training induced changes in skeletal muscle fibers.

Fiber Type	% Distribution			
	Before[1]	After	Before[2]	After
STR	41	43	57.9	56.5
FTR	37	42[*]	26.4	31.5[+]
FTW	19	14[*]	9.2	3.4[+]

[*]Significantly different from before, p<0.001.
[+]Significantly different from before, p<0.005.
[1]Data taken from Andersen and Henriksson, 1977b.
[2]Data taken from Ingjer, 1979.

1970). The fiber type composition pre- and post-training from two regions of the gastrocnemius muscle are presented in Table 5-3.

Further insights into fiber type adaptation to aerobic training can be gained from Luginbuhl and coworkers (1984). Female rats were subjected to a 10-week training program to determine the influence of intense interval training on fiber type composition of various muscles in the hindlimb. Measurements were taken in the soleus, plantaris, red vastus lateralis, and white vastus lateralis muscles. The fiber composition of the soleus and white vastus lataralis did not change with training although the activity of citrate synthase increased by 18% and 106% respectively, demonstrating a training effect. Prior to training, 7.5% of the plantaris fibers and 8.5% of the red vastus lateralis fibers were STR. After training, the percentages increased to 14.3 and 22.1. The FTR and FTW fiber count remained constant in the plantaris but shifted in the red vastus lateralis. Initially 11.1% of this muscle was FTR fibers and 64.4% FTW. Post-training values were 20.9% FTR and 53.5% FTW.

The method for determining fiber type used by Luginbuhl et al. was different from the traditional method of classification done by histochemical analysis of myosin ATPase. In spite of the methodological differences, however, a change in the fiber type profile of the plantaris and red vastus lateralis muscles was demonstrated whereas no change occurred in the soleus or white vastus lateralis. This is interesting because citrate synthase activity increased in all of the muscles (range 18 to 106%). These data infer that an increase in aerobic enzyme capacity is not necessarily correlated with changes in fiber type composition.

Along this line of thinking, other researchers (Gollnick et al., 1973) have shown that aerobic exercise 1 hour/day, 4 days/week at 75 to 90% of $\dot{V}O_2$ max will increase the activities of succinate dehydrogenase 95% and PFK 117% without any change in fiber composition of the vastus lateralis muscle.

The results from the various studies presented suggest that a fiber type transformation may occur in response to aerobic exercise training, but that the nature and degree of that response could be depend-

Table 5-3. Training-induced changes in fiber type distribution of the red and white regions of the gastrocnemius.

Fiber Type	White Region		Red Region	
	Control	Trained	Control	Trained
STR	29 ± 3	$42 \pm 4^*$	48 ± 4	$64 \pm 4^*$
FTR	3 ± 1	2 ± 1	16 ± 2	12 ± 3
FTW	68 ± 4	$56 \pm 4^*$	36 ± 4	$24 \pm 3^*$

Values are means ± SEM.
*Significantly different from control, $p < 0.05$.

ent upon the intensity of the training protocol and/or the original fiber type population of the exercised muscle.

Fiber Type Response to Anaerobic Exercise Training

Very little evidence exists to suggest that high-intensity exercise training that taxes anaerobic glycolysis will alter the fiber type distribution within the trained muscle. Jacobs and coworkers (1987) have found a small increase in the number of FTR fibers of the vastus lateralis muscle following "sprint training" on a cycle ergometer. Their subjects trained 2 to 3 times per week by performing 2 to 6 bouts of 15 second and 30 second cycle sprinting. Training of the glycolytic pathway was evidenced when phosphofructokinase (PFK) activity rose 16% ($P<0.05$) following training. The percent FTR fibers increased in the trained group from 31.9 + 8.0 to 39.1 + 8.0% ($p<0.008$). However, there was no significant change in any other fiber type. The authors suggest a concomitant decrease occurred in the percent of STR fibers (57.7 + 16.6 to 48.3 + 9.3%), but this change was not supported statistically ($p<0.09$).

In an earlier study, Costill and associates (1979) trained the vastus lateralis muscle of men for 7 weeks with isokinetic strength exercises. The 30 second exercise bouts of maximal work used in this study taxed primarily anaerobic glycolysis because of the elevated muscle lactate concentrations seen during exercise (0.9 mmol/kg wet weight at rest, 19.4 mmol/kg wet weight during exercise). Elevated levels of phosphorylase and PFK also indicated an anaerobic training effect on the glycolytic pathway. However, there was no change in fiber type distribution within the muscle.

A recent study by Baker and Hardy (1989) using high-intensity canoeing training of the latissimus dorsi muscle also failed to show a change in muscle fiber composition due to training. Male subjects trained 3 days/week for 9 weeks with a canoeing ergometer. Each workout consisted of 10 repetitions of 1 to 3 minutes. Successful training was demonstrated by an 82% hypertrophy in the FT muscle fibers, but there was no change in fiber type distribution.

The exercise training protocol in these studies varied greatly with the intervals of sprint bouts ranging from 15 seconds to 3 minutes. Until further information directs us otherwise, we must conclude that anaerobic training that taxes the glycolytic pathways does not induce an alteration in muscle fiber type composition.

Fiber Type Response to Heavy Resistance Training

In a 1975 study by Thorstensson, Sjodin, and Karlsson, four moderately trained males were sprint trained for a period of 8 weeks. The training consisted of repetitive 5 second sprinting bouts on a motor-driven treadmill 3 to 4 days/week. The training protocol elicited a 36% increase in creatinephosphokinase (CPK) activity ($p < 0.01$), a 30% increase in ATPase activity ($p < 0.05$), and a 20% increase in myokinase activity ($p < 0.05$) all indicative of ATP-PC derived energy production. (Myokinase is an enzyme that catalyzes the interconversions among ATP, ADP, and AMP.) The heavy energy demand placed on the ATP-PC system did not elicit a change in fiber type distribution of the vastus lateralis muscle.

Again in 1976 Thorstensson's group looked at the fiber type response to training. This time, progressive strength training was performed 3 times/week for 8 weeks by healthy males. Myokinase activity in the vastus lateralis increased only 7.8% whereas CPK and PFK activity remained the same. The authors conclude that no change occurred in fiber composition following strength training. Costill's group (1979) came to a similar conclusion in their study when the 6 second maximal exercise bouts proven to heavily tax the ATP-PC energy systems failed to elicit a change in fiber type distribution.

Contrary to the above findings, there is support for a shift in fiber type distribution following heavy resistance training. Gonyea and Ericson (1976) have designed a unique system for weight training cats that produces muscular strength gains as well as hypertrophy. This system of training was used to study the contractile properties and fiber composition in skeletal muscle after heavy resistance training (Gonyea & Bonde-Petersen, 1978). Six cats were trained to lift weights for a period of 10 to 61 weeks. Following training, there was a significant reduction in FTR fibers (29 to 20%) in the exercised palmaris longus of the trained cats when compared to a control group of cats. In accordance with the reduction in FTR fibers, there was an increase in FTW fibers in the same trained muscles (45 to 58%). The data become difficult to interpret in light of the fact that the same trained muscles showed a significant increase in time to peak tension and half-relaxation time. The researchers suggest that as the fibers in the palmaris longus undergo hypertrophy there are alterations in their contraction properties.

Other examples of fiber type conversions in trained muscle have recently been presented. Twenty-four women completed a 20-week heavy resistance training program for the lower extremity. Results of histochemical analysis showed that FTR fibers increased from 32.5 to 39.3% whereas FTW fibers decreased from 16.2 to 2.7% ($p < 0.05$; Staron et al., 1989). In another study, the percentage of STR fibers in the deep rectus femoris of rats decreased from $16.8 + 0.9$ to $11.9 + 1.4\%$ in response to heavy resistance training (Yarsheski, Lemon, & Gilloteaux, 1990). Some of these data suggest the possibility for alterations in fiber type distribution following training of the ATP-PC energy systems, but no definite conclusions can be made at this time.

FIBER TYPE TRANSFORMATION OR FIBER SPLITTING?

Most of the studies reviewed thus far reported hypertrophy to some degree in the fibers of exercise-trained muscles. The extent of hypertrophy is about 40% for ST fibers and roughly 80 to 90% for FT fibers (Prince, Hikida, & Hagerman, 1976). There are only two possible ways for a muscle to hypertrophy. One is by increasing the size of the fibers within the muscle, and the other is by increasing the number of fibers within the muscle. Along the same line of thinking, a specific fiber type can constitute a larger portion of a given muscle after training by two mechanisms. One is by reproducing itself in order to increase its number in proportion to the other fiber types (fiber splitting). The other is by transforming some of the existing fibers into the fiber type in question (fiber transformation). As it is generally accepted that muscles hypertrophy with training, we will not talk about hypertrophy per se, but rather will focus our attention on fiber type transformation and splitting while keeping in mind that hypertrophy can occur under either of these conditions.

Fiber Type Transformation

Some of the most revered investigations into the transformation of muscle fiber type were performed over 30 years ago by Buller, Eccles, and Eccles (1960). These investigators surgically divided and cross-innervated nerves to fast and slow muscles. Thus, motoneurons formerly innervating the fast muscle regeneratively innervated the slow muscle, and vice versa for the motoneurons of the slow muscle. The muscles used in these experiments were the soleus (slow) and the flexor digitorum longus (FDL, fast) of kittens. Cross-innervation produced an acceleration of the contraction of the soleus muscle reinnervated by FDL nerve fibers and a slowing of the contraction of the FDL muscle reinnervated by soleus nerve fibers. These alterations in speed of contraction were manifest in both the contraction and half-relaxation times (Table 5-4). In addition, the stimulus interval for a contraction midway between the twitch and maximum tetanus was reduced from 57 to 28 milliseconds for the FDL-innervated soleus and extended from 25 to 65 milliseconds for the soleus-innervated FDL. For some reason, fiber transformation was not complete because further experiments revealed that the transformed FDL remained faster than a normal soleus, whereas a transformed soleus remained slower than a normal FDL. In spite of incomplete transformation, these data indicate that transformation of one fiber to another is possible and that nerve innervation has a strong influence on fiber type differentiation.

This information leads one to wonder if fiber type contractile properties are due to neural innervation or just frequency of motoneural

Table 5-4. Contraction and half-relaxation times for control
and cross-innervated muscles.

	Contraction Time (msec)	Half-Relaxation Time (msec)
Control soleus	60	62
Experimental soleus (FDL-innervated)	42	45
Control FDL	33	32
Experimental FDL (soleus-innervated)	59	67

discharge. For example, motoneurons innervating ST muscles discharge at a frequency of 10 to 20/second, whereas those innervating FT muscle discharge at a rate of 30 to 60/second. If frequency of motoneural activity influences contraction time, then it should be possible to change ST fibers into FT and vice versa by controlling frequency of motoneuron discharge. This possibility was tested in some classical experiments performed by Salmons and Vrbová (1969).

The tenotomized soleus muscle of rabbits was stimulated artificially at a frequency of 40 hertz for a period of 15 to 20 days. The result was a faster soleus muscle. Conversely, when rabbit tibialis anterior and extensor digitorum longus, or cat flexor hallucis longus muscles were stimulated at a rate of 10 hertz for 2 to 6 weeks, they became slower. Once again the transformation in either direction was incomplete. These data show that frequency of neural discharge is a key to fiber type transformation and differentiation.

Salmons and Streter (1976) performed experiments in which long-term electrical stimulation was used to mimic as well as oppose the effects of cross-innervation. The rabbit peroneal nerve (fast) was connected to the soleus in a manner similar to previous cross-innervation experiments. Half the cross-innervated muscles were stimulated electrically at a rate of 10 hertz. The muscles that were only cross-innervated became faster when compared to controls, whereas those that were cross-innervated as well as stimulated became slower than controls. In addition to changing the contractile properties of the muscle, ATPase activity and calcium uptake by the sarcoplasmic reticulum were altered relative to changes in contraction time.

Some support for the reversible nature of fiber type transformation with exercise training has been provided by Jansson, Sjodin, and Tesch (1987). These researchers had athletes train both aerobically and anaerobically and took muscle biopsies after each type of training. After anaerobic training, the athletes had a lower percentage of STR fibers and a higher percentage of type IIc fibers. (Type IIc fibers have been identified as intermediate fibers in transition from FT to ST or vice versa.) The authors suggest that anaerobic training caused a conversion of STR fibers to type IIc, and that during aerobic training the conversion was in the opposite direction. One weakness of this study was that no control values were reported prior to either training schedule.

Guth and Yellin (1971) suggest that muscle cells undergo continual alterations in adaptation to functional demand and that classification of fiber types merely reflects a muscle's constitution at a given moment in time. They also point out that histochemical analysis of enzyme activity in muscle fibers can give rise to more classifications than the traditional three. With this in mind, only a more detailed analysis of fiber type characteristics than the histochemical examination may be necessary to determine if fiber type transformation actually occurs.

Rubinstein and associates (1978) demonstrated in a unique experiment the transformation of muscle fibers due to chronic stimulation. Specific antibodies against fast (AF) and slow (AS) muscle myosins of rabbits were prepared. Examinations of normal fast and slow muscle revealed that individual fibers within the muscle reacted with either AF or AS but not both. In other words, each fiber contains either a fast or slow myosin, but not both.

The rabbit peroneal nerve (fast) was then stimulated at 10 hertz for up to 8 weeks. Two possibilities for transformation within the muscle existed. If each individual fiber were committed to the synthesis of only one myosin type, then transformation of a fast muscle to a slow muscle would be demonstrated by degeneration of some fast fibers and new synthesis of slow fibers. Regardless of the stage of transformation of the muscle, individual fibers would stain with either AF or AS, but not both. However, if transformation involves a change in gene expression within existing fibers to synthesize a different myosin type, then fibers staining with both AF and AS should be found at some point during transformation.

After 3 weeks of stimulation, most of the fibers of the peroneus longus muscle (fast) stained with AF. (Some fibers did not stain.) At 4.5 weeks, most fibers stained with both AF and AS. At this stage of transformation, the fibers staining only with AS were probably slow fibers before stimulation. Those that stained with AS and AF were probably fast fibers in the process of transformation. By 8 weeks of stimulation, all the fibers stained uniformly with AS, and none stained with AF. According to these findings, transformation was a result of a switch from expression of fast myosin genes to the expression of slow myosin genes within the same fiber. These findings do not preclude the possibility of fiber type splitting as an additional mechanism for altering a muscle's fiber composition.

Exercise-induced changes in myosin expression of rat vastus lateralis muscle were reported by Green and coworkers (1984). Rats were endurance trained for 15 weeks on a rodent treadmill. Training caused an increase in the expression of slow myosin light chains, a decrease in fast myosin light chains, and a decrease in parvalbumin content of the deep vastus lateralis muscle (Table 5-5). Training also reduced the amount of 115,000-Mr calcium-pumping ATPase protein with a concomitant elevation in the 30,000-Mr peptide (Table 5-5). All of these changes are indicative of a fiber type transformation from fast to slow.

Fiber Type Splitting

Traditional thinking has said that the fiber content of skeletal muscle is determined at birth and that muscle growth occurs solely by hypertrophy of existing fibers. We have just seen that fiber composition of a muscle may change through fiber type transformation. Let's now see if any evidence indicates that fiber composition of a muscle may change through cell proliferation.

Moss and Leblond (1970) used the electron microscope to reveal the existence of two types of nuclei within the basement membrane of fibers from growing muscle. The first type of nuclei was directly associated with the myofibril-containing cytoplasm. These were called *true* nuclei. The second type of nuclei were surrounded by cytoplasm that was not associated with the myofibrils. These nuclei were separated from the contractile proteins by an intracellular space and were called satellite nuclei. These satellite nuclei were shown to be able to synthesize DNA (deoxyribonueleic acid), which synthesis precedes mitosis. The authors hypothesized that satellite cells associated with muscle fibers undergo mitosis and subsequently function as myoblasts, developing into new muscle fibers.

Ten years later Salleo and associates (1980) gave further support for this hypothesis when they found satellite cells developing into new muscle fibers during compensatory hypertrophy of rat skeletal muscle. Excising the gastrocnemius muscle of the rat will cause compensatory hypertrophy of the synergistic plantaris muscle. This operative procedure was performed on a group of rats and the hypertrophied

Table 5-5. Exercise-induced fiber transitions in myosin, parvalbumin, and sarcoplasmic reticulum peptides.

(moles/mole myosin)	Control	Exercise Trained
Myosin Light Chain		
1s	0.25 ± 0.15	0.61 ± 0.03*
1f	1.28 ± 0.11	1.13 ± 0.06*
3f	0.47 ± 0.14	0.26 ± 0.05*
Parvalbumin (mg/g protein)	27.3 ± 6.0	Non-detectable
Sarcoplasmic reticulum peptide ratio (115,000-Mr/30,000-Mr)	3.2 ± 1.1	$1.2 \pm 0.3^{+}$

Values are means ± SD.   Control vs. exercise trained, *$p<0.05$, +$p<0.001$.

plantaris muscles removed 15, 30, and 60 days post surgery. Hypertrophy was demonstrated by a 60, 77, and 94% increase in muscle weight found at 15, 30, and 60 days respectively. Electron microscopy revealed satellite cells that enlarged and became free from their connective sheaths. These satellite cells moved further away from their parent cells and subsequently underwent cell division. Rows of these newly divided cells formed elongated structures with a common sheath. These structures developed into new muscle fibers.

The animal model for exercise-induced hypertrophy developed by Gonyea and Ericson (1976) was used again in 1977 by Gonyea, Ericson, and Bonde-Petersen to demonstrate muscle fiber splitting induced by weight lifting in cats. Cats were trained to move a weighted bar with their right forelimb a specific distance for food. Following several weeks of training the flexor carpi radialis muscle (FCR) was removed. Significant hypertrophy was seen in the exercised muscle. The trained FCR showed a 19.3% increase in total number of fibers over the untrained FCR of the opposite limb. There was no significant alteration in the distribution of fibers due to training. The authors concluded that the increase in fiber number was due to fiber splitting which was of parallel magnitude in both the ST and FT fibers.

Gonyea repeated the same training experiment in 1980 with a few modifications. This time two groups of trained cats were used. One group weight trained with a low resistance (0.71 kg) and the other group with a high resistance (1.28 kg). After 34 weeks of training, the FCR muscle of the trained and untrained forelimb was removed in addition to the FCR of a control group of cats that didn't exercise. Some of the data generated are shown in Table 5-6. There was a 20.5% increase in the number of muscle fibers of the exercised FCR. This hyperplasia was only evident, however, in the high-resistance group. There was significant hypertrophy of the oxidative fibers in the low-resistance group, whereas the high-resistance group had hypertrophy in all fiber types. Gonyea concludes that the increases in muscle diameter seen with training are due both to hypertrophy of existing fibers and to formation of new fibers through fiber splitting. Similar results were produced again in 1986 by Gonyea's group using a different method for determining fiber type.

Skeletal muscle fiber splitting without accompanying hypertrophy was demonstrated by Ho et al. (1980). Rats trained to lift weights by standing upright in response to a stimulus were used in this study. With training, an 11% increase occurred in the number of fibers per cross-sectional area of the adductor longus muscle. Each fiber type, however, atrophied in response to the training protocol. The authors offer no explanation for this atrophy, when one would expect fiber-type hypertrophy from such a training protocol. Expressing fiber number per

Table 5-6. Comparison of FCR muscles between control and weight-trained cats.

Fiber Diameter (μm)	Control	Low Resistance	High Resistance
STR	37.1 ± 0.1	41.6 ± 0.3*	40.4 ± 0.2*
FTR	40.4 ± 0.2	41.6 ± 0.4*	44.8 ± 0.3*
FTW	51.6 ± 0.2	51.5 ± 0.4	57.1 ± 0.4*
Total Fiber #	7528 ± 532	7817 ± 405	9055 ± 420*

Values are means ± SEM.
*Significantly different from control, $p < 0.005$.

cross-sectional area of the muscle may not be the best indication of fiber type splitting, but the authors also present some data from electron microscopic examination that suggest longitudinal splitting of muscle fibers.

One of the criticisms against the notion of fiber type splitting in response to exercise is that all of the evidence for muscle fiber proliferation has come from animal research. The human research supporting fiber type splitting within exercised muscle has been either descriptive in nature (Edstrom & Ekbolm, 1972; Gollnick et al., 1972; Prince, Hikida, & Hagerman, 1976; Tesch, Thorsson, & Kaiser, 1984) or only suggestive due to alterations in fiber composition of trained muscle (Alway et al., 1989; Andersen & Henriksson, 1977b; Ingjer, 1979; Jacobs et al., 1987; Larsson & Tesch, 1986; Simoneau et al., 1985; Yarsheski, Lemon, & Gilloteaux, 1990). On the other hand, plenty of research suggests no change in fiber composition or number within a muscle resulting from training (Baker & Hardy, 1989; Costill et al., 1979; Larsson & Tesch, 1986; MacDougall et al., 1984; Tesch & Karlsson, 1985; Thorstensson et al., 1976; Thorstensson, Sjodin, & Karlsson, 1975). At this time it seems prudent to say that splitting of fiber types can occur in animal muscle under conditions of heavy training, but strong evidence for proliferation of muscle fibers in human muscle remains to be seen.

EXERCISE TRAINING AND CAPILLARIZATION

Although the adaptive response in capillary supply to exercise-trained muscle is not well documented, it does not seem to be as controversial as the subject of fiber type adaptation. The descriptive studies indicate that endurance athletes have increased capillarization when compared to untrained controls, and that weight lifters/power lifters have decreased capillarization. For example, Brodal, Ingjer, and Hermansen (1976) studied capillary supply to skeletal muscle fibers in endurance-trained and untrained men. Mean fiber diameters were not significantly different between groups, indicating that if a difference in capillary supply was found, it would not be due to hypertrophy diluting the existing supply. The capillarization expressed as capillaries per fiber was about 40% greater in the endurance-trained athletes (2.49 + 0.08) compared to the untrained men (1.77 + 0.10). The number of capillaries per mm² of muscle was also about 40% greater in the endurance athletes (821 + 28 vs. 585 + 40).

Heavy resistance training resulting in significant fiber hypertrophy seems to dilute the concentration of capillaries within the trained muscle. Schantz (1982) found that the mean number of capillaries per fiber in heavy-resistance trained subjects was 95% greater than untrained subjects. However, the number of capillaries per cross-sectional area of the muscle was the same for both groups. Bell and Jacobs (1990) have produced the same type of data for male and female body builders.

Tesch, Thorsson, and Kaiser (1984) also found that muscle hypertrophy decreased capillarization, but that it was expressed a little differently than the previous studies suggested. In this study, capillary supply in the vastus lateralis muscle of weight lifters/power lifters was compared to that of endurance athletes as well as nonathletes. The results are shown in Table 5-7. When capillarization was expressed as capillaries per fiber, the endurance athletes had about 50% more capillaries than both the weight lifters/power lifters and the nonathletes. The difference among groups was magnified when capillarization was expressed as capillaries per mm² of muscle. These data seem to infer that endurance training results in increased capillarization, whereas heavy resistance training results in decreased capillarization.

The above studies are descriptive in nature, and thus it cannot be determined if the differences in capillarization among the groups were inherent or a result of training. Andersen and Henriksson (1977a), on the other hand, have shown that endurance training increases capillary density and that capillarization increases equally with respect to each fiber type. Subjects in their study trained 40 minutes/day, 4 days/week, for 8 weeks on a bicycle ergometer at about 80% of $\dot{V}O_2$ max. The training protocol caused a 20% increase in capillary density expressed as

Table 5-7. Capillary supply in the vastus lateralis muscle of weight lifters/power lifters, endurance athletes, and nonathletes.

Group	Capillaries/Fiber	Capillaries/mm²
Weight lifters/Power lifters	2.06 ± 0.74	199 ± 29[+]
Endurance athletes	3.11 ± 0.73[*]	401 ± 61[+]
Nonathletes	2.16 ± 0.34	306 ± 29[+]

Values are means ± SD.

[*]Significantly different from the nonathletes, $p < 0.01$.
[+]Significantly different from other groups, $p < 0.01$.

capillaries per cross-sectional area of the vastus lateralis muscle. Capillaries per fiber increased by 47% due to training. Capillary supply to each fiber type increased to about the same degree, whether expressed as capillaries in contact with each fiber (31 to 40%) or capillary contact relative to fiber area (10 to 13%).

Ingjer (1979) also found increases in capillarization in the vastus lateralis after untrained women were subjected to 24 weeks of running at 50 to 90% of $\dot{V}O_2$ max for 45 minutes, 3 days a week. The average number of capillaries per muscle fiber increased 29% going from 1.39 ± 0.06 to 1.79 ± 0.08 ($p<0.005$). Capillaries per mm^2 increased by approximately 26% going from 348 ± 29 to 438 ± 31 ($p<0.005$). As shown in Table 5-8, the amount of capillaries around each fiber, as well as capillaries around each fiber relative to fiber size, increased with training. Ingjer, unlike Anderson and Henriksson, found that increased capillarization due to training was fiber type specific, being greatest for the STR fibers and least for the FTW fibers. Others (Klausen, Anderson, & Pelle, 1981) have similarly found increases in capillary supply to endurance-trained muscle.

TRAINING-INDUCED CHANGES IN MITOCHONDRIAL SIZE AND NUMBER

As aerobic metabolism occurs inside the mitochondria, it seems logical that muscle mitochondria should respond to aerobic exercise training. Research in the late 60s and early 70s has well established that the concentration of mitochondrial protein increases with aerobic or endurance exercise. The nature of this training response is an increase in both the size and number of mitochondria within the trained muscle (Barnard, Eggerton, & Peter, 1970; Davies, Packer, & Brooks, 1981; Gollnick & King, 1969; Holloszy, 1967; Holloszy & Oscai, 1969; Hoppeler et al., 1973).

The most notable paper on this topic was published by Holloszy in

Table 5-8. Changes in capillarization of the vastus lateralis muscle following endurance training.

Fiber Type	CA		CA/mm²	
	Before	After	Before	After
STR	4.1 ± 0.2*	5.0 ± 0.2*[+]	1.07*	1.27*[+]
FTR	3.4 ± 0.2*	4.2 ± 0.2*[+]	0.99*	1.13*[+]
FTW	2.3 ± 0.2*	2.7 ± 0.1*[+]	0.84*	0.92*[+]

CA = capillaries around each fiber. CA/mm² = capillaries around each fiber relative to fiber area ($\mu m^{-2} \times 10^{-3}$). Values are means ± SEM.
*Significantly different from other fiber types within the same group, $p<0.005$.
[+]Significantly different from the value before training, $p<0.01$.

1967. The aerobic exercise training protocol developed for rats in this study has become a classic and is worth detailing. Male rats were trained to run on a motor-driven treadmill designed for rodents. Motivation was provided by a shock grid at the rear of the treadmill. Animals learned to avoid being shocked by keeping pace with the treadmill belt. The belt was set at an 8% incline and the animals were exercised 5 days/week. Initially, the rats ran for 10 minutes, twice daily, 4 hours apart, at 22 meters/minute. This workload was progressively increased so that by the end of 12 weeks the animals were running continuously for 120 minutes at 31 meters/minute, with twelve 30-second sprints at 42 meters/minute interspersed every 10 minutes throughout the workout. Animals maintained this final work level until sacrificed. This training protocol caused a 57% increase in mitochondrial protein within the gastrocnemius muscle (Figure 5-3).

Holloszy and Oscai did another exercise training study in 1969 that produced a 59% increase in mitochondrial protein within the trained gastrocnemius muscle. Eighteen weeks of treadmill running also produced a 30% increase in mitochondrial protein within the gastrocnemius and plantaris muscles of exercised guinea pigs (Barnard, Eggerton, & Peter, 1970). Then in 1981 in a detailed analysis of the mitochondrial adaptation to endurance training, Davies, Packer, and Brooks reported that mitochondrial protein content increased in the hindlimb muscles

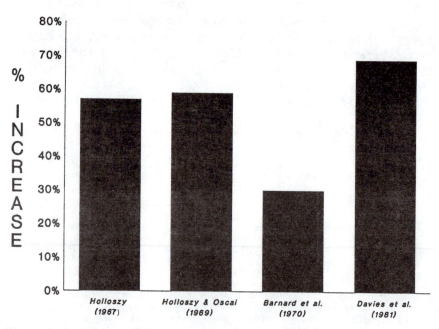

Figure 5-3. Training-induced increases in mitochondrial protein.

of aerobically-trained rats by 69%. The data from these four animal studies has been simplified and presented in Figure 5-3. Thus, it appears that chronic aerobic training augments mitochondrial protein content in muscle by approximately 50 to 60%.

The mechanism behind the manifested increase in mitochondrial protein content of endurance-trained muscle could be expressed by multiplying the number of mitochondria within the muscle or by increasing the size of existing mitochondria. Gollnick and King (1969) have shown that the number of mitochondria in endurance-trained rat gastrocnemius muscle is 50 to 100% greater than in untrained muscle, whether expressed relative to muscle cross-sectional area or sarcomere number (Figure 5-4). These investigators also noted that the trained mitochondria appeared to be enlarged with more densely packed cristae when compared to the untrained mitochondria, although they did not quantify the size difference.

Research from Hoppeler and associates (1973) helps clarify the concept of exercise-induced enlargement of muscle mitochondria. This investigative team compared the mitochondria from the vastus lateralis muscle of trained orienteers to that of sedentary men and women.

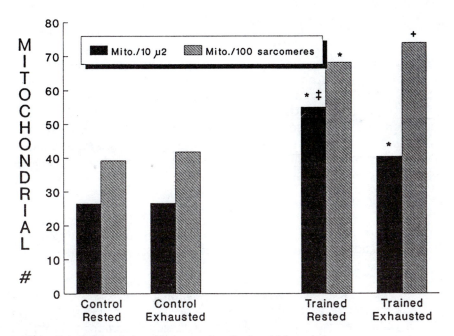

Figure 5-4. Training-induced increases in mitochondrial number.
  *Significantly different from controls, $p < 0.05$.
  ⁺Significantly different from controls, $p < 0.01$.
  ‡ Significantly different from trained exhausted, $p < 0.05$.

They found that the volume density of the interfibrillar mitochondria in the orienteers was 47% higher than in the sedentary males and 44% higher than in the sedentary females. The surface area of these mitochondria was also greater in the orienteers than in the males (28%) and females (74%). The volume density of the subsarcolemmal mitochondria in the orienteers was 3.2 and 2.1 times greater than that of the sedentary males and females respectively. Finally, the surface of the mitochondrial cristae in the orienteers was greater than in the untrained men and women (62% and 133%, respectively).

Exercise-induced changes in mitochondrial size and number were found to be fiber type specific as well as training specific in a recent paper by Takekura and Yoshioka (1989). Male rats were either sprint trained (anaerobic) or endurance trained (aerobic) on a motor-driven treadmill. Single fibers from the soleus and extensor digitorum longus muscles were dissected and analyzed. The mitochondrial volume in the STR fibers of the endurance-trained group was significantly ($p < 0.01$) greater than that of the control and sprint-trained groups. However, in the FTR fibers the mitochondrial volume was significantly ($p < 0.01$) greater in the sprint-trained group than in the other two groups. Significantly ($p < 0.01$) more mitochondria were also observed in the FTR fibers of the sprint-trained group compared to the endurance-trained group and controls.

One does not expect mitochondrial adaptations to heavy resistance training because the aerobic energy pathways are not taxed during this type of exercise. Indeed, morphometric analysis of the triceps brachii before and after 6 weeks of heavy resistance training revealed a 26% reduction in mitochondrial volume density and a 25% reduction in the mitochondrial volume to myofibrillar volume ratio (MacDougall et al., 1979). This implies that heavy resistance training leads to a dilution in mitochondrial content in muscle due to hypertrophy of the myofibrills.

CONCLUSIONS

The following conclusions can be made with respect to muscle ultrastructural adaptations to exercise training.

1. A relationship exists between fiber type distribution of a muscle and type of exercise training. This relationship may be exercise-induced as well as inherited.
2. Aerobic exercise training could alter the fiber composition of a muscle by increasing the relative proportion of aerobic fibers within the muscle.

3. Anaerobic exercise training that taxes primarily the glycolytic energy pathways will not alter a muscle's fiber type distribution.
4. Anaerobic exercise training that taxes primarily the ATP-PC energy pathways will probably not alter the fiber composition of the trained muscle.
5. A more detailed analysis for classifying fiber types other than histochemistry may be necessary before definitive results can be obtained relative to exercised-induced changes in fiber type distribution.
6. Muscle hypertrophy due to training can result from enlargement and/or hyperplasia of individual fibers.
7. Muscle fibers can proliferate in some animal species, but evidence for proliferation of human muscle fibers is lacking.
8. Aerobic exercise training can increase capillary supply to the trained muscle, whereas heavy resistance training may reduce capillary supply.
9. Aerobic exercise training causes an increase in the size and number of mitochondria of the trained muscle, whereas heavy resistance training can dilute the mitochondrial content because of myofibrillar hypertrophy.
10. The ultrastructural adaptations in muscle to chronic exercise training are relative to fiber type as well as being dependent upon intensity of work, length of training period, and original fiber composition of the muscle.

REFERENCES

Alway, S.E., Grumbt, W.H., Gonyea, W.J., & Stray-Gundersen, J. (1989). Contrasts in muscle and myofibers of elite male and female bodybuilders, *J. Appl. Physiol.*, 67(1): 24-31.

Andersen, P. & Henriksson, J. (1977a). Capillary supply of the quadriceps femoris muscle of man: adaptive response to exercise, *J. Physiol.*, 270: 677-690.

Andersen, P. & Henriksson, J. (1977b). Training induced changes in the subgroups of human type II skeletal muscle fibres, *Acta Physiol. Scand.*, 99: 123-125.

Baker, S.J. & Hardy, L. (1989). Effects of high intensity canoeing training on fibre area and fibre type in the latissimus dorsi muscle, *Br. J. Sports Med.*, 23(1): 23-26.

Barnard, R.J., Eggerton, V.A., & Peter, J.B. (1970). Effect of exercise on skeletal muscle I. Biochemical and histochemical properties, *J. Appl. Physiol.*, 28(6): 762-766.

Bell, D.G. & Jacobs, I. (1990). Muscle fibre area, fibre type & capillarization in male and female body builders, *Can. J. Sports Science*, 15(2): 115-119.

Brodal, P., Ingjer, F., & Hermansen, L. (1976). Capillary supply of skeletal muscle fibers in untrained and endurance trained men, *Acta Physiol. Scand. Suppl.*, 440: 296.

Buller, A.J., Eccles, J.C., & Eccles, R.M. (1960). Interactions between motoneurons and muscles in respect of the characteristic speeds of their responses, *J. Physiol.*, 150: 417-439.

Costill, D.L., Coyle, E.F., Fink, W.F., Lesmes, G.R., & Witzmann, A. (1979). Adaptations in skeletal muscle following strength training, *J. Appl. Physiol.*, 46(1): 96-99.

Davies, K.J.A., Packer, L., & Brooks, G.A. (1981). Biochemical adaptation of mitochondria, muscle and whole-animal respiration to endurance training, *Arch. Biochem. Biophys.*, 209(2): 539-554.

Edstrom, L. & Ekbolm, B. (1972). Differences in sizes of red and white muscle fibres in vastus lateralis of musculus quadriceps femoris of normal individuals and athletes. Relation to physical performance, *Scand. J. Clin. Lab. Invest.*, 30: 175-181.

Gollnick, P.D., Armstrong, R.B., Saltin, B., Saubert C.W., IV, Sembrowich, W.L., & Shepherd, R.E. (1973). Effect of training on enzyme activity and fiber composition of human skeletal muscle, *J. Appl. Physiol.*, 34(1): 107-111.

Gollnick, P.D., Armstrong, R.B., Saubert, C.W., IV, Piehl, K., & Saltin, B. (1972). Enzyme activity and fiber composition in skeletal muscle of untrained and trained men, *J. Appl. Physiol.*, 33(3): 312-319.

Gollnick, P.D. & King, D.W. (1969). Effect of exercise and training on mitochondria of rat skeletal muscle, *Am. J. Physiol.*, 216(6): 1502-1509.

Gonyea, W. (1980). Role of exercise in inducing increases in skeletal muscle fiber number, *J. Appl. Physiol.*, 48(3): 421-426.

Gonyea, W. & Bonde-Petersen, F. (1978). Alterations in muscle contractile properties and fiber composition after weight-lifting exercise in cats, *Exp. Neurol.*, 59: 75-84.

Gonyea, W. & Ericson, G.C. (1976). An experimental model for the study of exercise-induced skeletal muscle hypertrophy, *J. Appl. Physiol.*, 40: 630-633.

Gonyea, W., Ericson, G.C., & Bonde-Petersen, F. (1977). Skeletal muscle fiber splitting induced by weight-lifting exercise in cats, *Acta Physiol. Scand.*, 99: 105-109.

Gonyea, W., Sale, D.G., Gonyea, F.B., & Mikesky, A. (1986). Exercise induced increases in muscle fiber number, *Eur. J. Appl. Physiol.*, 55: 137-141.

Green, H.J., Klug, G.A., Reichmann, H., Seedorf, U., Wiehrer, W., & Pette, D. (1984). Exercise-induced fibre type transitions with regard to myosin, parvalbumin, and sarcoplasmic reticulum in muscles of the rat, *Pflugers Arch.*, 400: 432-438.

Guth, L. & Yellin, H. (1971). The dynamic nature of the so-called "fiber types" of mammalian skeletal muscle, *Exp. Neurol.*, 31: 277-300.

Ho, K.W., Roy, R.R., Tweedle, C.D., Heusner, W.W., Van Huss, W.D., & Carrow, R.E. (1980). Skeletal muscle fiber splitting with weight-lifting exercise in rats, *Am. J. Anat.*, 157: 433-440.

Holloszy, J.O. (1967). Biochemical adaptations in muscle, *J. Biol. Chem.*, 242(9): 2278-2282.

Holloszy, J.O. & Oscai, L.B. (1969). Effect of exercise on α-glycerophosphate dehydrogenase activity in skeletal muscle, *Arch. Biochem. Biophys.*, 130: 653-656.

Hoppeler, H., Luthi, P., Claassen, H., Weibel, E.R., & Howald, H. (1973). The ultrastructure of the normal human skeletal muscle, *Pflugers Arch.*, 344: 217-232.

Ingjer, F. (1979). Effects of endurance training on muscle fibre ATP-ase activity, capillary supply and mitochondrial content in man, *J. Physiol.*, 294: 419-432.

Jacobs, I., Esbjornsson, M., Sylven, C., Holm, I., & Jansson, E. (1987). Sprint training effects on muscle myoglobin, enzymes, fiber types, and blood lactate, *Med. Sci. Sports Exerc.*, 19(4): 368-374.

Jansson, E., Sjodin, B., & Tesch, P. (1978). Changes in muscle fibre type distribution in man after physical training, *Acta Physiol. Scand.*, 104: 235-237.

Klausen, K., Anderson, L.B., & Pelle, I. (1981). Adaptive changes in work capacity, skeletal muscle capillarization and enzyme levels during training and detraining, *Acta Physiol. Scand.*, 113: 9-16.

Larsson, L. & Tesch, P.A. (1986). Motor unit fibre density in extremely hypertrophied skeletal muscles in man, *Eur. J. Appl. Physiol.*, 55: 130-136.

Luginbuhl, A.J., Dudley, G.A., & Staron, R.S. (1984). Fiber type changes in rat skeletal muscle after intense interval training, *Histochemistry*, 81: 55-58.

MacDougall, J.D., Sale, D.G., Alway, S.E., & Sutton, J.R. (1984). Muscle fiber number in biceps brachii in bodybuilders and control subjects, *J. Appl. Physiol.*, 57(5): 1399-1403.

MacDougall, J.D., Sale, D.G., Moroz, J.R., Elder, G.C.B., Sutton, J.R., & Howald, H. (1979). Mitochondrial volume density in human skeletal muscle following heavy resistance training, *Med. Sci. Sports Exerc.*, 11(2): 164-166.

Moss, F.P. & Leblond, C.P. (1970). Nature of dividing nuclei in skeletal muscle of growing rats, *J. Cell Biol.*, 44: 459-462.

Prince, F.P., Hikida, R.S., & Hagerman, F.C. (1976). Human muscle fiber types in power lifters, distance runners and untrained subjects, *Pflugers Arch.*, 363: 19-26.

Rubinstein, N., Mabuchi, K., Pepe, K., Salmons, S., Gergely, J., & Streter, F. (1978). Use of type-specific antimyosins to demonstrate the transformation of individual fibers in chronically stimulated rabbit fast muscles, *J. Cell Biol.*, 79: 252-261.

Salleo, A., Anastasi, G., LaSpada, G., Falzea, G., & Denaro, M.G. (1980). New muscle fiber production during compensatory hypertrophy, *Med. Sci. Sports Exerc.*, 12(4): 268-273.

Salmons, S. & Streter, F.A. (1976). Significance of impulse activity in the transformation of skeletal muscle type, *Nature*, 263: 30-34.

Salmons, S. & Vrbová, G. (1969). The influence of activity on some contractile characteristics of mammalian fast and slow muscles, *J. Physiol.*, 201: 535-549.

Schantz, P. (1982). Capillary supply in hypertrophied human skeletal muscle, *Acta Physiol. Scand.*, 114: 635-637.

Simoneau, J.-A., Lortie, G., Boulay, M.R., Marcotte, M., Thibault, M.-C., & Bouchard, C. (1985). Human skeletal muscle fiber type alteration with high-intensity intermittent training, *Eur. J. Appl. Physiol.*, 54: 250-253.

Staron, R.S., Malicky, E.S., Leonardi, M.J., Falke, J.E., Hagerman, F.C., Dudley, G.A. (1989). Muscle hypertrophy and fast fiber type conversions in heavy resistance-trained women, *Eur. J. Appl. Physiol.*, 60: 71-79.

Takekura, H. & Yoshioka, T. (1989). Specific mitochondrial responses to running training are induced in each type of rat single muscle fibers, *Jap. J. Physiol.*, 39: 497-509.

Tesch, P.A. & Karlsson, J. (1985). Muscle fiber types and size in trained and untrained muscles of elite athletes, *J. Appl. Physiol.*, 59(6): 1716-1720.

Tesch, P.A., Thorsson, A., & Kaiser, P. (1984). Muscle capillary supply and fiber type characteristics in weight and power lifters, *J. Appl. Physiol.*, 56(1): 35-38.

Thorstensson, A., Hulten, B., von Doblen, W., & Karlsson, J. (1976). Effect of strength training on enzyme activities and fibre characteristics in human skeletal muscle, *Acta Physiol. Scand.*, 96: 392-398.

Thorstensson, A., Sjodin, B., & Karlsson, J. (1975). Enzyme activities and muscle strength after "sprint training" in man, *Acta Physiol. Scand.*, 94: 313-318.

Yarsheski, K.E., Lemon, P.W.R., & Gilloteaux, J. (1990). Effect of heavy-resistance exercise training on muscle fiber composition in young rats, *J. Appl. Physiol.*, 69(2): 434-437.

6

EXERCISE-INDUCED ADAPTATIONS IN THE ATP-PC ENERGY SYSTEM

As mentioned earlier, the driving force behind biological adaptation is a disruption in homeostasis. When an energy system of the body is disrupted, it attempts to overcome that disrupted state or "stress" by making the necessary changes to bring back homeostasis. The chronic "stress" of exercise training will bring about many adaptations in the energy-producing pathways allowing a new level of homeostasis to be achieved. The principle of "specificity of training" must be kept in mind as we discuss the adaptations that occur in each of the energy-producing pathways. In other words, the biochemical adaptations that occur in response to exercise training will be specific to the type of training performed. For example, heavy resistance training that taxes primarily the ATP-PC energy system will result in metabolic adaptations specific to that system. Although this principle of specificity of training will generally apply to each energy system, it must be remembered that the metabolic pathways are not completely independent of each other. For the sake of simplicity in presentation, Chapters 6 through 8 of this book will focus separately upon specific adaptations in the ATP-PC, glycolytic, and aerobic energy pathways.

ENZYMATIC ADAPTATION TO VERY INTENSE EXERCISE TRAINING

The most critical factor to exercise performance is the production of energy to sustain that exercise. Therefore, the primary indication of biochemical adaptation in a metabolic pathway is an increase in activity of the regulatory enzymes of that metabolic pathway. One of the first experiments to demonstrate an enzymatic adaptation to very intense exercise training was performed in 1975 by Thorstensson and coworkers. The training stimulus imposed upon 4 healthy males in this research was a series of 5 second sprints repeated 20 to 40 times, 3 to 4 days/week, for 8 weeks. Muscle biopsies from the lateral portion of the vastus lateralis were taken before and after the training period. Enzyme activity increased for myosin ATPase (30%, $p<0.05$), myokinase (20%, $p<0.05$), and creatine phosphokinase (36%, $p<0.01$). Lactate dehydrogenase activity did not change with this type of training.

A year later Thorstensson's group (1976) used a strength training protocol to study enzyme activity and fiber characteristics in muscle. Fourteen male subjects performed "squat" exercises 3 times a week in which 3 sets of 6 repetitions with maximal weight were completed each exercise session. This type of training did not produce any significant changes in ATPase or creatine phosphokinase (CPK) activities and only produced a 7.8% increase in myokinase (MK) activity ($p<0.05$) of the vastus lateralis muscle.

Around this same period of time researchers in the Soviet Union were heavily involved in the biochemistry of sport. An excellent review paper by Yakovlev (1975) provides us with much information pertinent to the biochemical adaptations to training in skeletal muscle. With respect to very intense exercise training at maximal power, the Soviets have found skeletal muscle ATPase activity to increase by 55% in response to training, but they have failed to see any significant changes in CPK or lactate dehydrogenase (LDH) activities.

A few years later, a group of researchers from Sweden strength-trained 10 women daily for 5 weeks using one-leg exercises consisting of 3 periods of 10 maximal voluntary knee extensions (Krotkiewski et al., 1979). Comparisons pre- to post training revealed a 36% increase in MK activity and a 58% increase in LDH activity in muscle biopsy samples from the vastus lateralis.

More recently, Tesch and associates (1989) have performed a descriptive analysis of the enzyme activity in the different fiber types of heavy-resistance-trained athletes. Tissue samples from the vastus lateralis muscle of elite olympic weight lifters and body builders were compared to those of sedentary men. LDH activity for the athletes averaged 62% higher in the FT fibers and 50% higher in the ST fibers when compared to the sedentary men. It is interesting to note here that although the LDH activity for all the men was much lower in the ST fibers than the FT fibers, the ST fibers still responded to the training stimulus by increasing their LDH activity. In contrast, MK activity in the ST fibers did not respond to training, whereas it did in the FT fibers by a magnitude of about 40%.

In opposition to the findings previously discussed, 7 weeks of isokinetic strength training failed to alter enzyme activities for LDH, CPK, or MK (Costill et al., 1979). However, the isokinetic strength training did elevate phosphofructokinase (PFK) activity by 7% in the trained muscle of these subjects. In addition to the already mentioned enzymatic adaptations in the anaerobic pathways, cytochrome oxidase, succinate dehydrogenase, and aspartate aminotransferase activities have been shown to increase in response to very intense exercise training (Yakovlev, 1975). In contrast, other researchers have found that citrate synthase activity was 26 to 67% lower in the FT fibers and that 3-hydroxyacyl CoA dehydrogenase activity was 17 to 32% lower in the ST fibers of strength-trained athletes when compared to untrained men (Tesch, Thorsson, Essen-Gustavsson, 1989). Figure 6-1 summarizes the magnitude of *anaerobic* enzymatic augmentation seen in the various studies that *have* demonstrated an exercise-induced increase in enzyme activity following very intense exercise training.

In spite of the discrepancies in the literature, it seems safe to conclude that very intense exercise training is most likely to increase the activity of myosin ATPase, MK, and LDH. Failure to induce consistent enzymatic responses in all of the investigations could be due to differences in training protocol. On the other hand, the adaptations in the glycolytic or aerobic pathways seen in some of the experiments could be due to differences in training protocol or cross training effects.

VERY-HEAVY-EXERCISE-INDUCED CHANGES IN SUBSTRATE USE AND STORAGE

If exercise performance is dependent upon energy production and energy production dependent upon enzyme capacity as well as

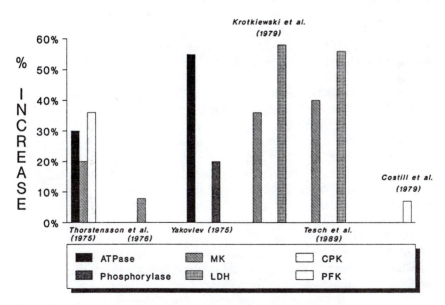

Figure 6-1. Anaerobic enzyme adaptation to very intense exercise training.

substrate availability, then logically one of the adaptive mechanisms to exercise training may be an alteration in substrate storage or utilization. Although Thorstensson, Sjodin, and Karlsson (1975) found that ATPase, MK, and CPK increased with very intense training, they found no changes in the content of ATP or PC stored in the exercise-trained muscles. On the other hand, others find adequate support for the notion that a muscle's ability to store and utilize metabolic fuel is increased with very-intense-exercise training (MacDougall et al., 1977; Yakovlev, 1975).

Reports from the Soviet Union have shown that exercise training at maximal power output increases resting muscle glycogen content 38%, and PC content 15 to 30% (Yakovlev, 1975). In addition, the maximal capacity for the muscle tissue to utilize specific substrates for fuel increased with very intense training. For example, lactate production increased between 18 and 55% following training while the capacity to oxidize pyruvate increased 60%. Tissue respiratory capacity was also elevated by 30 to 70% due to training at maximal power output.

Researchers in Canada have gone beyond investigating the biochemical adaptations to heavy resistance training to look at the effects of muscle use and disuse on metabolic adaptation (MacDougall et al., 1977). Nine male subjects strength-trained the biceps brachii for 5 months with heavy resistance exercises in addition to having the biceps brachii of the opposite arm immobilized for 5 weeks. Strength training increased the content of glycogen in the biceps brachii by 66% in contrast to a 40% reduction in glycogen concentration following muscle disuse. PC stores were elevated by 22% in the trained muscle compared to a 25% PC reduction in the immobilized muscle. In addition, the heavy resistance training caused an 18% increase in ATP storage, a 39% increase in creatine content, and a calculated augmentation in the intracellular adenosine pool of about 23%. The data from these studies looking at metabolite storage and utilization following intense exercise training have been summarized and presented in Figure 6-2.

Some insights into the reasons why these biochemical adaptations to chronic exercise training occur can be gained by studying the effects of a single exercise bout on muscle metabolism. Recently, the muscle metabolic changes occurring during intense, heavy resistance exercise were monitored in the vastus lateralis muscle of 9 strength-trained athletes (Tesch, Colliander, & Kaiser, 1986). Each athlete completed an exercise regimen comprised of 5 sets of 6 to 12 repetitions executed to muscle failure of front squats, back squats, leg presses, and knee extensions. Muscle biopsies were taken before and immediately following the exercise bout. Figure 6-3 illustrates what happened to the muscle content of various metabolites involved in anaerobic energy production. As seen from the figure, the intense exercise de-

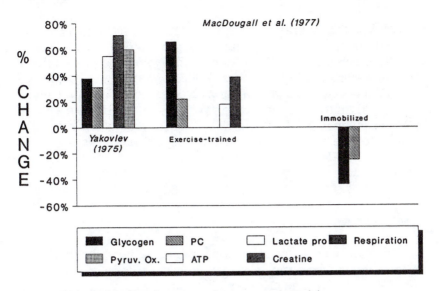

Figure 6-2. Metabolic adaptations to very intense exercise training.

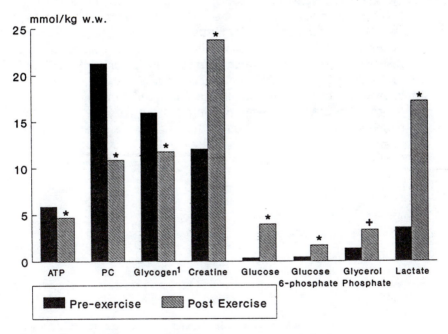

Figure 6-3. Metabolic changes following a single intense exercise bout.
  *Significantly different from pre-exercise, p<0.01.
  ⁺Significantly different from pre-exercise, p<0.05.
  [1]glycogen content = mmol/100 grams wet weight.

creased ATP, PC, and glycogen stores significantly, and glucose and glycolytic intermediates rose dramatically during the exercise bout. The authors concluded that high intensity, heavy resistance exercise is associated with a high rate of energy utilization through phosphagen (ATP, PC) breakdown and activation of glycogenolysis. This augmented metabolic flux through the anaerobic pathways in response to a single exercise bout may be the reason why other investigators found that chronic exercise training at a very high intensity produces enzymatic and metabolic adaptations in both the ATP-PC and glycolytic energy systems.

CONCLUSIONS

The following conclusions can be made relative to the biochemical adaptations that occur in skeletal muscle following a period of chronic exercise training at a very high intensity.

1. Exercise training at a level near maximal power output will increase the trained muscle's capacity for anaerobic energy production.
2. Regulatory enzymes in both the ATP-PC and glycolytic pathways can increase their maximal activity following training at maximal power output. The enzymes most likely to increase their activity in response to this type of training are: myosin ATPase, MK, LDH, CPK, PFK, and phosphorylase.
3. In order to accomodate the muscle's "new" enzymatic capacity for energy production following training, intermediary metabolites are more highly concentrated in the resting muscle. These elevated storage levels of metabolites include ATP, PC, creatine, and glycogen.

REFERENCES

Costill, D.L., Coyle, E.R., Fink, W.F., Lesmes, G.R., & Witzmann, F.A. (1979). Adaptations in skeletal muscle following strength training. *J. Appl. Physiol.*, 46(1): 96-99.
Krotkiewski, M., Aniansson, A., Grimby, G., Bjorntorp, P., & Sjorstom, L. (1979). The effect of unilateral isokinetic strength training on local adipose and muscle tissue morphology, thickness, and enzymes. *Eur. J. Appl. Physiol.*, 42:271-281.
MacDougall, J.D., Ward, G.R., Sale D.G., & Sutton, J.R. (1977). Biochemical adaptation of human skeletal muscle to heavy resistance training and immobilization. *J. Appl. Physiol.*, 43(4): 700-703.
Tesch, P.A., Colliander, E.B., & Kaiser, P. (1986). Muscle metabolism during intense, heavy-resistance exercise. *Eur. J. Appl. Physiol.*, 55: 362-366.
Tesch, P.A., Thorsson, A., & Essen-Gustavsson, B. (1989). Enzyme activities of FT and ST fibers in heavy-resistance trained athletes. *J. Appl. Physiol.*, 67(1): 83-87.

Thorstensson, A., Hulten, B., von Dublen, W., & Karlsson, J. (1976). Effect of strength training on enzyme activities and fiber characteristics in human skeletal muscle. *Acta Physiol. Scand.*, 96:392-398.

Thorstensson, A., Sjodin, B., & Karlsson, J. (1975). Enzyme activities and muscle strength after "sprint training" in man. *Acta Physiol. Scand.*, 94: 313-318.

Yakovlev, N.N. (1975). Biochemistry of sport in the Soviet Union: beginning, development, and present status. *Med. Sci. Sports*, 7(4): 237-247.

7

GLYCOLYTIC ADAPTATIONS TO EXERCISE

Intense exercise lasting more than 20 to 30 seconds, but less than 3 to 4 minutes, will be supported primarily by the resynthesis of ATP via anaerobic glycolysis. We will learn from this chapter what biochemical adaptations occur following intense exercise training that increase one's capacity for glycolytic energy production.

GLYCOLYTIC ENZYME RESPONSES TO ANAEROBIC TRAINING

The most important enzyme regulating glycolytic energy production is phosphofructokinase (PFK). Thus it seems logical that anaerobically trained muscle should have a higher activity of PFK than untrained or even aerobically trained muscle. However, this does not seem to be the case according to the descriptive analysis performed on muscle biopsies taken from several groups of athletes and nonathletes (Gollnick et al., 1972). When comparing the PFK activity in the deltoid and vastus lateralis muscles of weight lifters to that of various endurance athletes, Gollnick et al. found no training effect upon PFK (Figure 7-1). Any definite conclusion is difficult from this data because one can only assume that the weight lifters were training primarily the anaerobic pathways and that the endurance athletes were training primarily the aerobic pathways.

More specific information relative to the enzymatic adaptations to anaerobic training comes from the Soviet Union (Yakovlev, 1975). Exercise training at high speed, which typically taxes the glycolytic pathway, increased enzyme activity for myosin ATPase, creatine phosphokinase (CPK), phosphorylase, hexokinase (HK), PFK, pyruvate kinase (PK), and lactate dehydrogenase (LDH) when compared to untrained muscle (Figure 7-2).

A training program designed to stress the glycolytic energy producing pathways was employed by Costill et al. (1979) in an attempt to elucidate the metabolic adaptations to anaerobic exercise training.

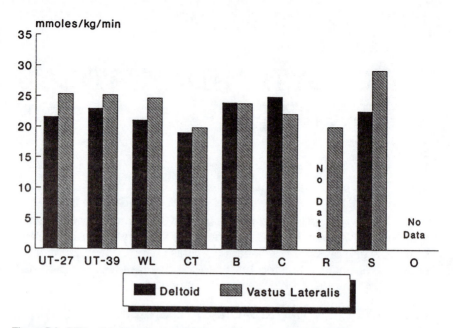

Figure 7-1. PFK activity in muscles of various athletes and nonathletes. UT-27 and UT-39 represent untrained groups with an average age of 27 and 39 years respectively. WL = Weight lifters. CT = Cross-trained. B = Bicyclists. C = Canoeists. R = Runners. S = Swimmers. O = Orienteers.

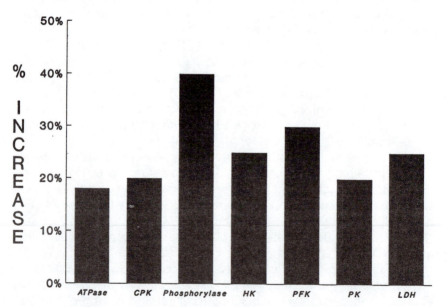

Figure 7-2. Increases in anaerobic enzyme activity following high-speed training.

The 7-week program consisted of 30-second maximal exercise bouts of the knee extensors. Support for the fact that anaerobic glycolysis was stressed during this training protocol comes from the tremendous increase in muscle lactate content seen during the exercise (0.9 mmol/kg, rested; 19.4 mmol/kg, exercised). The training of the glycolytic system increased enzyme levels for myokinase (MK), CPK, PFK, and phosphorylase (Figure 7-3) but not to the extent reported by Yakovlev (Figure 7-2).

Other researchers who have demonstrated an increase in PFK activity with glycolytic exercise training showed activity levels augmented to the same extent as seen previously (Costill et al., 1979; Yakovlev, 1975). For example Fournier et al. (1982) reported a 21% increase in PFK activity, Jacobs et al. (1987) a 16% increase in PFK levels, and Simoneau et al. (1987) a 14 to 34% increase. In the latter study, in addition to PFK increases, HK activity was elevated 33% above control levels following 15 weeks of high-intensity intermittant training.

Insights into the fiber-type specificity of glycolytic exercise training can be gained from the recent work of Takekura and Yoshioka (1990). In their study, male rats were exercise-trained on a rodent treadmill for 16 weeks. The training protocol consisted of interval running for 45 seconds at a speed of 85 meters/minute, 10 times at 2.75 second intervals. All training was performed 5 days/week. Enzyme activity was determined in the soleus and extensor digitorum longus (EDL)

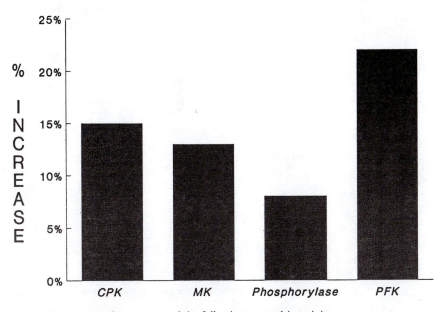

Figure 7-3. Increases in enzyme activity following anaerobic training.

muscles as well as individual muscle fibers for CPK, LDH, PFK, PK, succinate dehydrogenase (SDH), and malate dehydrogenase (MDH). The sprint training caused a 30% decrease in CPK activity and an 18% decrease in LDH activity within the soleus muscle. In contrast, CPK activity was reduced by only 14% in the EDL whereas PFK (27%), PK (53%), and SDH (44%) were all elevated. As the soleus contains primarily STR fibers and the EDL contains primarily FTR and FTW fibers, the increase in glycolytic enzymes in the EDL could be a reflection of heavy recruitment upon the fast-twitch fibers during the sprint-training protocol. This idea is further upheld when the enzyme data for individual fibers are analyzed (Figure 7-4). It is interesting to note that the activity of the glycolytic enzymes (PFK, LDH, and PK) increased in the FTR and FTW fibers following sprint training, but not in the STR fibers (Figure 7-4). On the other hand, the activity of the aerobic enzymes (SDH and MDH) increased in all of the fiber types. These data indicate that the glycolytic adaptations to anaerobic exercise training are fiber-type specific, occurring only in the fibers best suited for anaerobic energy production.

As was expected, anaerobic exercise training that primarily stressed the glycolytic energy-producing pathways caused an increase in glycolytic enzyme activity, particularly PFK. Although this type of training wouldn't be expected to elevate aerobic enzyme activity, most of the investigators that reported increased glycolytic enzyme activity also saw elevated aerobic enzyme levels. For example, high-speed training caused SDH, citrate synthase (CS), cytochrome oxidase (CO), and NADH

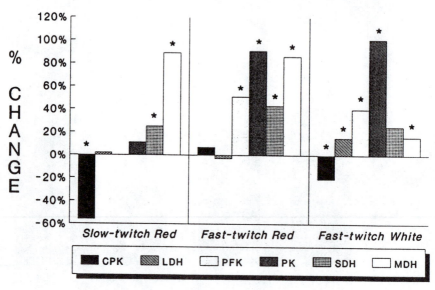

Figure 7-4. Enzyme changes in muscle fiber types following sprint training.
*Significant change, p<0.05.

reductase to become more active (Figure 7-5; Yakovlev, 1975). In fact, the high-speed training had a more pronounced effect on these aerobic enzymes than it did upon the glycolytic enzymes (compare Figures 7-5 and 7-2.). Simoneau's group (1987) also saw that high-intensity intermittant training elevated aerobic enzymes to a greater extent than glycolytic enzymes (6). Oxoglutarate dehydrogenase (26%), MDH (53 to 68%), and 3-hydroxyacyl CoA deyhydrogenase (52 to 103%) activities increased proportionately more than HK (33%) and PFK (14 to 34%). Costill et al. (1979) found increases in MDH (14%) and SDH (11%) that were of a similar magnitude to their glycolytic enzyme changes (Figure 7-3), but not as dramatic as those reported by others (Simoneau et al., 1987; Takekura & Yoshioka, 1990; Yakovlev, 1975). Jacobs and co-workers (1987) also reported only small increases in both PFK (16%) and CS (12%) activities after glycolytic training. Finally, Takekura and Yoshioka (1990) saw increases in SDH and/or MDH in all three fiber types after sprint training. Although aerobic enzyme activity may increase with glycolytic training, the magnitude of increase will not be as dramatic as seen with aerobic training.

For example, 13 male subjects used one-legged bicycle exercise either to train one leg for endurance and the other for speed, one leg for speed while not training the other, or one leg for endurance while not training the other (Saltin et al., 1976). Training consisted of 5 work-

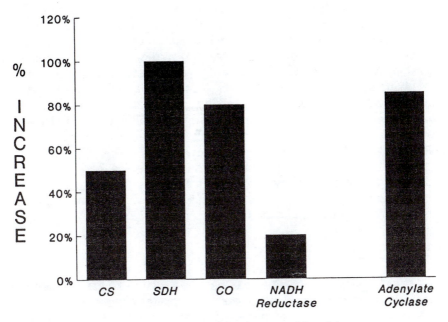

Figure 7-5. Elevations in aerobic enzymes following anaerobic training.

outs per week for 4 weeks at 75% $\dot{V}O_2$ max for endurance and 150% $\dot{V}O_2$ max for speed. SDH activity was elevated by 19% in the sprint-trained muscles and 33% in the endurance-trained muscles. Unfortunately, these investigators did not measure any glycolytic enzymes, so we cannot compare responses due to their training protocol on both aerobic and glycolytic enzyme activity. However, the readers can make their own conclusions by comparing the review presented in this chapter with that presented in Chapter 8.

An opposing view relative to sprint training and aerobic enzyme activity is put forth by Davies, Packer, and Brooks (1982). They found that sprint training did not affect the aerobic enzymes CO, pyruvate oxidase, palmitoyl-carnitine oxidase, or succinate oxidase. These authors suggest that sprint training does not affect aerobic enzyme capacity in spite of small increases in the capacity for aerobic metabolism.

SUBSTRATE USE AND STORAGE FOLLOWING GLYCOLYTIC EXERCISE TRAINING

Very intense anaerobic training of short duration was demonstrated in Chapter 6 to increase muscle concentration of ATP, PC, and glycogen. Intense anaerobic training of moderate duration such as speed training or intermittant sprint training also increases the concentration of ATP, PC, and glycogen in the muscle (Houston & Thompson, 1977; Yakovlev, 1975). Figure 7-6 shows that of these three substrates, glycogen concentration is augmented the most, followed by PC stores, and then ATP. Corresponding to the increased storage of glycogen in the muscle, peak blood lactate concentration post exercise is raised by 10 to 14% (Houston & Thompson, 1977; Jacobs et al., 1987). In addition, high-speed training increases the ability of the muscle to produce ATP as well as its capacity for glycolysis (Figure 7-7; Yakovlev, 1975). These biochemical adaptations to glycolytic exercise training all favor an accelerated rate of anaerobic energy production.

The capacity for aerobic energy production is also increased with high-speed training (Yakovlev, 1975). This increased aerobic capacity is manifested by a higher rate of cell respiration with a greater capacity to oxidize pyruvate, succinate, and palmitate (Figure 7-7).

CONCLUSIONS

The following conclusions can be made relative to the biochemical adaptations occurring in skeletal muscle after a chronic period of intense exercise training of moderate duration.

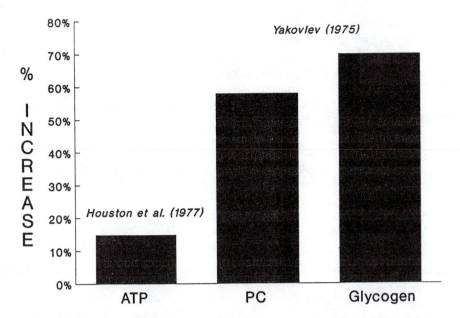

Figure 7-6. Changes in substrate storage following speed or intermittant sprint training.

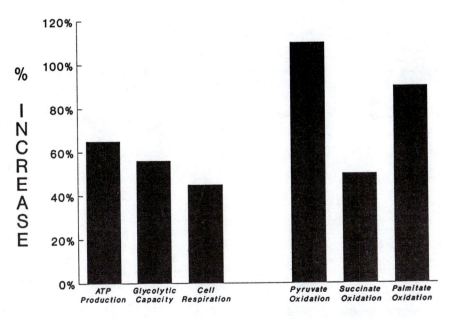

Figure 7-7. Effects of high-speed training upon the capacity to produce energy.

1. Anaerobic exercise training aimed at stressing the glycolytic pathway will increase the activity of the anaerobic enzymes by approximately 20 to 100%. These enzymes include myosin ATPase, CPK, HK, PFK, PK, LDH, and phosphorylase.
2. Anaerobic exercise training aimed at stressing the glycolytic pathway *may* increase activity of some aerobic enzymes. Those enzymes most likely to respond are CS, SDH, CO, MDH, and NADH reductase.
3. Glycolytic enzyme adaptation to sprint training may be fiber type specific, with the training response manifesting primarily in the fast-twitch fibers because of their heavier recruitment during this type of exercise.
4. Anaerobic exercise training aimed at stressing the glycolytic pathway will increase the concentration of stored ATP, PC, and glycogen within the resting muscle, with the largest adaptation seen for muscle glycogen.
5. Anaerobic exercise training aimed at stressing glycolytic energy production will increase the muscle's capacity for total ATP production, its capacity for glycolysis, and its capacity for oxidative metabolism.

REFERENCES

Costill, D.L., Coyle, E.F., Fink, W.F., Lesmes, G.R., & Witzmann, F.A. (1979). Adaptations in skeletal muscle following strength training. *J. Appl. Physiol.*, 46(1): 96-99.

Davies, K.J.A., Packer, L., & Brooks, G.A. (1982). Exercise bioenergetics following sprint training. *Arch. Biochem. Biophys.*, 215(1): 260-265.

Fournier, M., Ricci, J., Taylor, A.W., Ferguson, R.J., Montpetit, R.R., & Chaitman, B.R. (1982). Skeletal muscle adaptation in adolescent boys: sprint and endurance training and detraining. *Med. Sci. Sports Exer.*, 14(6): 453-456.

Gollnick, P.D., Armstrong, R.B., Saubert, C.W., IV, Piehl, K., & Saltin, B. (1972). Enzyme activity and fiber composition in skeletal muscle of untrained and trained men. *J. Appl. Physiol.*, 33(3): 312-219.

Houston, M.E. & Thomson, J.A. (1977). The response of endurance-adapted adults to intense anaerobic training. *Eur. J. Appl. Physiol.*, 36: 207-213.

Jacobs, I., Esbjornsson, M., Sylven, C., Holm, I., & Jansson, E. (1987). Sprint training effects on muscle myoglobin, enzymes, fiber types, and blood lactate. *Med. Sci. Sports Exerc.*, 19(4): 368-374.

Saltin, B., Nazar, K., Costill, D.L., Stein, E., Jansson, E., Essen, B., & Gollnick, P.D. (1976). The nature of the training response; peripheral and central adaptations to one-legged exercise. *Acta Physiol. Scand.*, 96: 289-305.

Simoneau, J.-A., Lortie, G., Boulay, M.R., Marcotte, M., Thibault, M.-C., & Bouchard, C. (1987). Effects of two high-intensity intermittant training programs interspaced by detraining on human skeletal muscle and performance. *Eur. J. Appl. Physiol.*, 56: 516-521.

Takekura, H. & T. Yoshioka (1990). Different metabolic responses to exercise training programmes in single rat muscle fibers. *J. Muscle Res. Cell Motil.* 11(2): 105-113.

Yakovlev, N.N. (1975). Biochemistry of sport in the Soviet Union: beginning, development, and present status. *Med. Sci. Sports*, 7(4): 237-247.

8

METABOLIC ADAPTATIONS FOLLOWING AEROBIC EXERCISE TRAINING

The biochemical adaptations to aerobic exercise training will be a little easier to define than those following anaerobic training because the aerobic pathways are more distinct than the anaerobic pathways (ATP-PC and glycolysis). Another distinguishing feature of aerobic metabolism is that fat can only be catabolized aerobically. This becomes significant because any stimulus that proves to affect fat-derived energy production will be perceived clearly as producing an aerobic adaptation. As fat, carbohydrate, and protein can all be catabolized aerobically, the scope of biochemical adaptation to aerobic exercise training is potentially greater than that for anaerobic training.

ADAPTATIONS IN AEROBIC ENZYME SYSTEMS

From a chronological standpoint, research into the enzymatic adaptations to aerobic exercise training preceded the research relating to the anaerobic adaptations by about 5 years. The premier scientist in this area of investigation is John O. Holloszy. Dr. Holloszy, along with his postdoctoral research fellows, discovered many of the enzymatic and metabolic adaptations occurring in muscle in response to aerobic exercise training. The first and most notable paper published on this topic was printed in 1967. The aerobic exercise training protocol developed in this study has proven to be very reliable for producing metabolic adaptations to aerobic exercise training in rat skeletal muscle. Male rats were trained to run on a motor-driven treadmill designed for rodents. Motivation was provided by a shock grid at the rear of the treadmill. Animals learned to avoid being shocked by keeping pace with the treadmill belt. The belt was set at an 8% incline and the animals were exercised 5 days/week. Initially, the rats ran for 10 minutes, twice daily, 4 hours apart, at 22 meters/minute. This workload was progressively increased so that by the end of 12 weeks the animals were running continuously for 120 minutes at 31 meters/minute, with twelve 30-second sprints at 42 meters/minute interspersed every 10 minutes throughout the workout. Animals maintained this final work level until sacrificed.

Tissue samples were taken from the soleus and gastrocnemius muscles for a sedentary group of rats as well as from an exercise-trained group. Enzyme activity was measured for various enzymes specifically associated with the electron transport system. Table 8-1 reveals the enzymatic changes that occurred in skeletal muscle following aerobic training. Cytochrome oxidase (CO) activity increased 62 to 81% as a result of training. Succinate oxidase (SO), which is involved in the transfer of electrons from succinate to coenzyme Q of the electron transport chain and links the oxidation of succinate to oxygen, increased 60 to 68%. Succinate dehydrogenase (SDH) was also increased following training (82%). NADH dehydrogenase and NADH cytochrome C reductase activities were elevated by 111% and 140% respectively. In addition to the enzymatic changes resulting from aerobic training, the trained muscles exhibited an 86% increase in cytochrome C content when compared to the untrained muscles. Holloszy also reported that the mitochondria from the exercise-trained muscles exhibited a high level of respiratory control and tightly coupled oxidative phosphorylation. This means that the increase in electron transport enzyme activity was associated with a rise in the muscle's capacity to produce ATP.

Two years later, Holloszy and Oscai (1969) published a paper where they again demonstrated that the rat training protocol Holloszy designed in 1967 could produce biochemical adaptations in the electron

Table 8-1. Respiratory enzyme capacity in aerobically-trained vs. untrained skeletal muscle.

Enzyme	Sedentary	Exercised
Cytochrome oxidase[1]		
Gastrocnemius	305 ± 15	551 ± 31*
Soleus	427 ± 16	691 ± 52*
Succinate oxidase[1]		
Gastrocnemius	73 ± 5	117 ± 8*
Soleus	95 ± 10	160 ± 8*
NADH dehydrogenase[2]		
Gastrocnemius	5.6 ± 0.6	11.8 ± 1/5*
NADH cytochrome C reductase[2]		
Gastrocnemius	0.25 ± 0.05	0.60 ± 0.09[+]
Succinate dehydrogenase[2]		
Gastrocnemius	8.3 ± 0.7	15.1 ± 1.4*

Values are means ± SEM.
*Exercised vs. sedentary, $p < 0.001$. [+]$p < 0.01$. [1]$\mu l\ O_2$/min/g. [2]μmoles/min/g.

transport chain. This time there was a 91% increase in CO activity and a 101% increase in cytochrome C content in the trained gastrocnemius muscle compared to untrained muscle.

In a third study coming from Holloszy's lab, cytochrome C content of the grastrocnemius muscle of treadmill-trained rats was elevated above control values by 102% (Holloszy et al., 1970). Enzyme activity within the citric acid cycle was determined, and aerobic training was found to have increased the activity of various enzymes by 34 to 101% (Figure 8-1). NAD-specific isocitrate dehydrogenase (IDH), which is the rate limiting enzyme in the citric acid cycle, was 90% more active after training than it was before. The importance of these findings is that unlike the electron transport chain, the enzymes related to the citric acid cycle do not increase in parallel during the adaptation of skeletal muscle to aerobic training. This suggests a change in mitochondrial composition in response to aerobic exercise training as well as an increase in citric acid cycle and electron transport enzymes.

Additional investigations into the exercise-induced adaptations to aerobic training repeatedly showed cytochrome C content to be increased (87%; Molé & Holloszy, 1970) along with the activities of IDH (95%; Molé & Holloszy, 1970), CO (91%; Oscai et al., 1971), and SO (71%, 66%; Molé & Holloszy, 1970; Oscai et al., 1971). The results of these early studies established quickly some of the major enzymatic adaptations to aerobic exercise training. Later research has only verified these

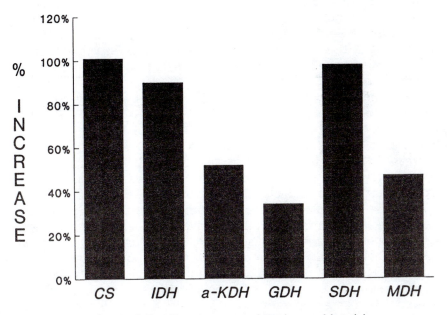

Figure 8-1. Elevations in citric acid cycle enzymes following aerobic training.

early findings. In fact, standard procedure now is for investigators to first verify their exercise-training protocol by manifesting an increase in cytochrome C content or activity of one of these aerobic marker enzymes before presenting any new findings relative to aerobic exercise-induced adaptations.

An example of this training verification comes in the next paper. This time, Oscai and Holloszy (1971) were investigating mitochondrial ATPase, creatine phosphokinase (CPK), and adenylate kinase (AK) responses to aerobic training. (The enzyme AK is important in liver and muscle where turnover of ATP is high. Its purpose is to maintain an equilibrium among AMP, ADP, and ATP. Oligomycin-sensitive ATPase was used as an indicator of F_1 activity or ATP synthesis in the mitochondria.) The rat training protocol was similar to that used previously (Holloszy, 1967). The concentration of cytochrome C was used as a marker for the electron transport chain. The content of cytochrome C in the gastrocnemius rose 115% in response to training, indicating a successful aerobic training effect. Mitochondrial oligomycin-sensitive ATPase activity increased by 76 to 113%, depending upon assay incubation procedures. However, the activity of mitochondrial CPK and AK were not affected by exercise training. The failure of CPK and AK to respond to training can be accepted as real and not just due to a faulty training protocol because the aerobic training protocol was verified by an increase in cytochrome C content. The increase in F_1 activity found by the authors is only further supported by the verification of the training procedures.

Further research into the enzymatic adaptations to aerobic training was done in 1971 (Molé, Oscai, & Holloszy). This research focused upon some of the enzymes specific to fatty acid metabolism. Rats were exercise-trained according to Holloszy's (1967) protocol and mixed muscle samples from the hindlimb were homogenized and used for enzyme measurements. Activity of ATP-dependent palmityl CoA synthetase increased 127% due to training, activity of carnitine palmityl-transferase (CPT) increased 89%, and palmityl CoA dehydrogenase increased 133% (Figure 8-2). These data suggest that in addition to the overall increase in aerobic enzyme capacity seen with training, the specific enzymes for fat metabolism also adapt to aerobic training.

Lactate accumulation in exercising muscle and blood is generally recognized as contributing to muscular fatigue by inactivating enzymes and by interfering with nerve stimulation and the contractile process (Bertocci & Gollnick, 1985; Brooks, 1988; Mainwood & Renaud, 1985). Any adaptation that results in decreased lactate accumulation would therefore prolong the onset of fatigue. Glutamate-pyruvate transaminase (GPT) is an enzyme that competes with lactate dehydrogenase (LDH) for glycolytically-produced pyruvate and causes the pyruvate

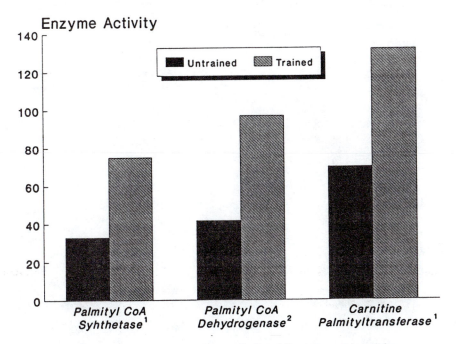

Figure 8-2. Enzyme activity for fat-specific metabolism following aerobic training.
[1]nmoles/min/g
[2]nmoles/min/g $\times 10^{-1}$

to be converted to alanine rather than lactate. Molé and coworkers
(1973) have demonstrated that the activity of GPT increases in rat
skeletal muscle following aerobic exercise training (Figure 8-3). This
increase in GPT activity may enhance exercise performance by di-
verting pyruvate away from lactate production.

Winder and associates (1974, 1975) studied the exercise-induced
adaptations occurring in the enzymes involved in ketone body utilization. Activity of 3-hydroxybutyrate dehydrogenase increased 159 to
471% in response to training, depending upon the fiber composition of
the muscle sampled. 3-ketoacid CoA transferase increased its activity
after training by a magnitude of 27 to 100%, while acetoacetyl CoA thio-
lase activity rose by 40 to 54%.

Others have reinforced these established enzymatic adaptations
to aerobic training in addition to adding new information to the growing pool of knowledge. For example, Green, Reichmann, and Pette
(1983) found that aerobic training increased the activities of 3-ketoacid
CoA transferase, CS, and GPT in both the deep and superficial portion
of the rat vastus lateralis muscle, as others have reported; but they also
found that the enzyme 3-hydroxyacyl CoA dehydrogenase (3-HAD)
was threefold more active in the superficial portion of the vastus latera-

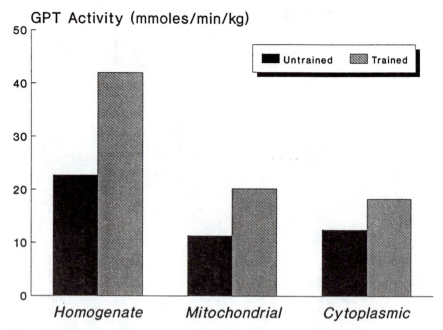

Figure 8-3. GPT activity in skeletal muscle following aerobic training.

lis muscle after 15 weeks of training, but only 56% more active in the deep vastus lateralis after training. Similarly, Davies, Packer, and Brooks (1981) reported increases in activity of the same magnitude as had previously been reported for citric acid cycle enzymes and electron transport enzymes. They have also found that cytochrome A content in trained muscle is 111% higher than in untrained muscle.

Aerobic Enzyme Adaptations Relative to Fiber Type Distribution

Most of the enzyme mesurements reported thus far have been made on muscle samples of a mixed fiber type distribution, with no attempt to differentiate adaptive responses among fiber types. As early as 1972, Baldwin and associates recognized the need to distinguish among fiber types when analyzing the biochemical adaptations to aerobic training. Initially, these researchers analyzed the fiber distribution in the rat muscle groups commonly used in biochemical research. Their fiber distribution pattern is presented in Table 8-2.

After their initial analysis, they determined cytochrome C content and the activities for CS, CO, CPT in the soleus (S), red vastus lateralis (RV) and white vastus lateralis (WV) muscles (Figure 8-4). They concluded that the capacity of all three fiber types for aerobic metabolism increases proportionately to the same extent.

Winder, Baldwin, and Holloszy (1974) also found similar increases

Table 8-2. Fiber type distribution of rat skeletal muscles.

Muscle	% STR	% FTR	% FTW
Soleus	96	4	—
Deep (red) vastus lateralis	30	70	—
Superficial (white) vastus lateralis	—	—	100

in CS activity and cytochrome C concentration among the different fiber types. However, they found dramatic differences in response among the fiber types for enzymes involved in ketone metabolism (Table 8-3).

Green, Reichmann, and Pette (1983) only compared enzyme activity in the RV and WV muscles following training but found a large difference in response between the red and white fibers (Table 8-4).

A more recent study (Takekura & Yoshioka, 1990) revealed that SDH and malate dehydrogenase (MDH) increased their activity in equivalent proportions in all three fiber types of rat skeletal muscle after aerobic training. In this study, male rats were exercise-trained on a rodent treadmill for 16 weeks. Training was increased to where the rats were running 120 minutes/day, 5 days/week at 40 meters/minute. Individual muscle fibers were analyzed for CPK, LDH, phosphofructokinase (PFK), pyruvate kinase (PK), SDH, and MDH. Figure 8-5 shows that although the aerobic enzymes SDH and MDH adapted to about the same extent, the glycolytic enzyme adaptation was fiber type specific. Greater reductions in glycolytic enzymes were found in the FTW fibers than in the FTR or STR ones (Figure 8-5).

Adaptations in NADH-Shuttle Enzymes

NAD^+ is reduced to NADH in the cytosol during glycolysis. Since NAD^+ content is limited, NADH produced during glycolysis must be reoxidized for glycolysis to continue. The anaerobic oxidation of NADH occurs when pyruvate is reduced to lactate. The aerobic oxidation of NADH occurs through the mitochondrial electron transport chain. Transport of NADH into the mitochondria is inhibited by the impermeability of the inner mitochondrial membrane to NADH. This barrier is bypassed by the transfer of reducing equivalents into the mitochondria via the malate-aspartate and the glycero-phosphate shuttles. As it is now well established that aerobic exercise training can result in an approximately twofold increase in the activities of the mitochondrial enzymes associated with the oxidation of NADH and succinate, it seems possible that the enzymes responsible for transferring cytosolic reducing equivalents into the mitochondria increase their activity in response to aerobic training. This possibility has been investigated (Holloszy, 1975;

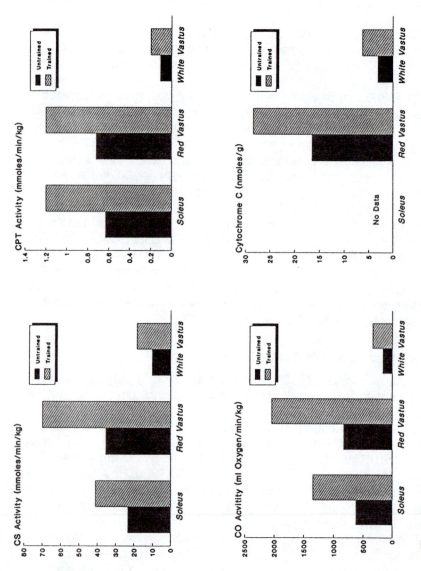

Figure 8-4. Fiber type specific responses to aerobic training.

Table 8-3. Fiber type specific changes in enzyme activity following aerobic training.

Enzyme	Soleus	% Increase RV	WV
Citrate synthase	104	88	86
3-Hydroxybutyrate dehydrogenase	159	471	—
3-Ketoacid CoA transferase	27	93	100
Acetoacetyl CoA thiolase	45	40	47

Holloszy & Oscai, 1969; Orlander et al., 1977; Schantz, Sjoberg, & Svendenhag, 1986).

Three different laboratories have looked at the effects of aerobic training upon α-glycerophosphate dehydrogenase activity (a key enzyme in the glycero-phosphate shuttle). All of these laboratories arrived at the same conclusion: α-glycerophosphate dehydrogenase activity does not change with aerobic training (Holloszy & Oscai, 1969; Orlander et al., 1977; Schantz, Sjoberg, & Svendenhag, 1986). This suggests that either the glycero-phosphate shuttle is not stressed to capacity during aerobic exercise or that cytosolic NADH entrance into the mitochondria is not a limiting factor in aerobic energy production during exercise.

Unlike the glycero-phosphate shuttle, the malate-aspartate shuttle does respond to training. Activity levels of aspartate transaminase (AT) and MDH were measured in both the cytosolic and mitochondrial fractions of aerobically-trained rat gastrocnemius muscle (Holloszy, 1975). Maximal activity of both enzymes was 35 to 96% higher following training (Figure 8-6).

Results from a later study (Schantz, Sjoberg, & Svendenhag, 1986) confirmed the findings of Holloszy (1975). Muscle biopsies from endurance-trained athletes were compared to those of untrained subjects. Measurements for MDH and AT in the cytosolic and mitochondrial fractions were taken. AT activity increased 46% ($p < 0.05$) in the cytosol and 49% ($p < 0.05$) in the mitochondria, while MDH activity was elevated by 48% ($p < 0.05$) in the mitochondria and 32% (not statistically significant) in

Table 8-4. Enzyme activity in the red and white portions of the vastus lateralis muscle following aerobic training.

Enzyme	% Increase RV	WV
Citrate synthase	67	247
3-Hydroxybutyrate dehydrogenase	56	319
Glutamate-Pyruvate transaminase	27	132

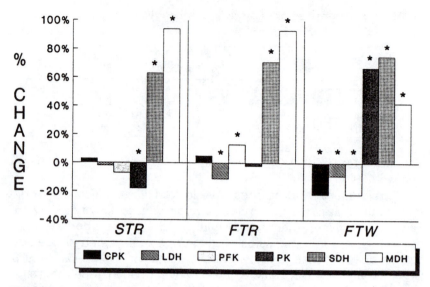

Figure 8-5. Enzyme changes specific to fiber types following aerobic training. *Significant change, $p < 0.05$.

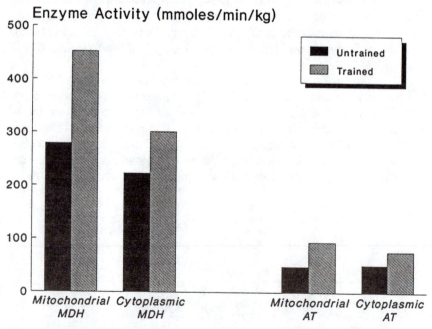

Figure 8-6. Malate-aspartate shuttle enzyme responses to aerobic training.

the cytosol. These two studies indicate that cytosolic NADH entrance into the mitochondria is a limiting factor in aerobic energy production, and that the malate-aspartate shuttle is stressed to maximal capacity during aerobic exercise.

A possible hypothesis for the training response in the malate-aspartate shuttle and not in the glycero-phosphate shuttle could be efficiency. The reducing equivalents from cytosolic NADH are transferred to FAD with a corresponding drop in energy potential in the glycero-phosphate shuttle. On the other hand, the reducing equivalents from cytosolic NADH are transferred to NAD^+ in the malate-aspartate shuttle. During exercise, when metabolic efficiency is critical, the malate-aspartate shuttle may be the primary system for the transport of reducing equivalents into the mitochondria. In contrast, the glycero-phosphate shuttle may be more active at rest.

GLYCOLYTIC ENZYME ADAPTATIONS TO AEROBIC TRAINING

As glucose and glycogen can be catabolized aerobically as well as anaerobically, certain adaptations in the glycolytic pathway could be resulting from aerobic training. Baldwin and associates investigated this possibility in 1973. Subjects for their study were male rats who were exercise-trained according to Holloszy's protocol (1967). Glycolytic enzyme activities were compared among the soleus (S), red vastus lateralis (RV), and white vastus lateralis (WV) muscles of exercise-trained and sedentary rats. The data are presented in Figure 8-7. It is interesting to see how the muscles representing the different fiber types responded differently to the training. The only consistent change in enzyme activity was seen with hexokinase (HK). However, HK response in the three muscles was of a different magnitude.

The glycolytic response in each muscle type was somewhat different for the other glycolytic enzymes. The S muscle, which has the lowest inherent capacity for glycolytic activity, showed significant increases in almost all of the glycolytic enzymes monitored. The WV, which has the highest inherent capacity for glycolytic work, showed the least amount of change in glycolytic enzyme activity. The puzzling result lies within the RV muscle's response. Because the RV muscle has a high capacity for both aerobic and glycolytic work, one would expect little change in the glycolytic enzyme profile of this muscle following aerobic training. However, most of the glycolytic enzymes decreased their activity following the aerobic training protocol. One possible explanation for this paradox relates back to fiber type transformations. The research in Chapter 5 has suggested that aerobic exercise training can transform the fiber type distribution of a muscle, and that the fibers most likely to transform are the FTR fibers. The FTR

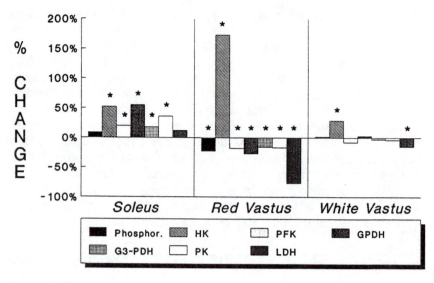

Figure 8-7. Glycolytic enzyme responses to aerobic training in 3 muscle types. *Significant change, $p < 0.05$.

fibers of the RV muscle may be undergoing a transformation towards the STR fibers, which would explain the decrease in glycolytic enzyme activity. This explanation is supported by the fact that even though the glycolytic enzyme activity for the RV muscle decreased in response to aerobic training, it was still two- to threefold higher than the elevated glycolytic activity of the trained S muscle.

Gollnick et al. (1972, 1973) reported conflicting findings relative to PFK activity in aerobically trained muscle. In their first study, they presented data on PFK activity for various endurance-trained athletes that indicated no adaptive response (see Figure 7.1; Gollnick et al., 1972). Then, a year later, they reported that subjects who trained for 5 months on a bicycle ergometer at 75% of their VO_2 max had PFK activity in the vastus lateralis muscle that was 117% higher than before training.

A decade later, Young and Holloszy (1983) reported that swim training increased HK activity in swim-trained rats by 22 to 40%. Phosphorylase and PK activity however, did not change with this swim-training protocol. In the same year, Green and coworkers (1983) reported a 40% increase in HK activity of the vastus lateralis muscle taken from treadmill-trained rats. They also reported that LDH, phosphorylase, glyceraldehyde 3-phosphate dehydrogenase, and fructose 1,6-diphosphatase activities were reduced following the training. Takekura and Yoshioka (1990) also reported small reductions in glycolytic enzymes in the three fiber types following aerobic exercise training

(Figure 8-5). Thus, it seems that the glycolytic enzyme response to aerobic exercise training is not as clear as that seen for the aerobic enzymes.

About the same time that exercise biochemistry was growing in the United States, it was also receiving much attention in the Soviet Union. Despite the difficulty acquiring and interpreting much of the Soviet research, a review paper printed in 1975 reveals some interesting parallels to what we have already established in this chapter (Yakovlev, 1975). The Soviets report that exercise of an aerobic nature increases muscle CPK, HK, AK, and phosphorylase activity. They also report elevations in CS, SDH, CO, and NADH reductase activities due to training (Figure 8-8).

ENZYME CHANGES IN HUMAN MUSCLE DUE TO AEROBIC TRAINING

The limited data available on the enzymatic adaptations to aerobic training in humans strongly supports that data found for animal muscle. Gollnick et al. (1972) provide us with some descriptive data comparing SDH activity in the deltoid and vastus lateralis muscles of athletes compared to nonathletes (Figure 8-9). Their data suggest that human muscle increases its SDH activity in response to aerobic training. In a

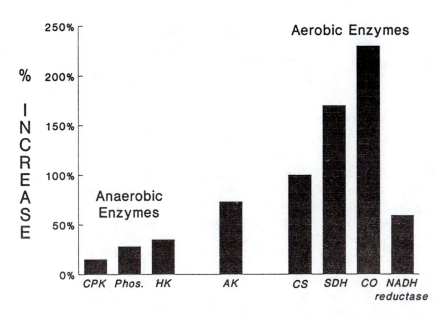

Figure 8-8. Enzyme response to aerobic exercise training. Phos. = phosphorylase. See text for other abbreviations.

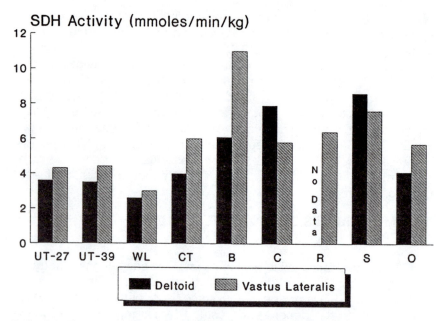

Figure 8-9. SDH activity in muscles of athletes and nonathletes. UT-27 and UT-39 represent untrained groups with an average age of 27 and 39 years respectively. WL = Weight lifters. CT = Cross-trained. B = Bicyclists. C = Canoeists. R = Runners. S = Swimmers. O = Orienteers.

followup study a year later, Gollnick's group (1973) found that aerobic training did indeed elevate SDH activity in aerobically-trained muscles. Six male subjects trained 1 hour/day, 4 days/week, for 5 months at 75% of their $\dot{V}O_2$ max. Muscle biopsy samples from the vastus lateralis muscle pre-and post training revealed a 95% increse in SDH activity due to the training.

Fournier and associates (1982) also found that aerobic training increased SDH activity in human muscle. A 3-month endurance training program increased SDH activity by 42% in the vastus lateralis muscle of adolescent boys. Furthermore, 6 months of detraining caused SDH activity to return back to pre-training levels. This shows that the enzymatic adaptations to training are reversible and not permanent.

Other enzyme changes in addition to SDH were measured by Evans and coworkers (1979). These investigators compared CPT, MDH, and SDH activities in the vastus lateralis of trained cyclists and the gastrocnemius of trained runners to the respective values for sedentary control subjects. The trained men had a higher capacity for aerobic metabolism, particularly fat oxidation which was manifest by elevated enzyme activity (Figure 8-10).

When Schantz and associates (1986) were investigating the effects

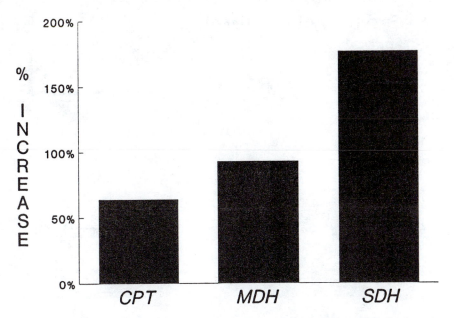

Figure 8-10. Elevated enzyme activity in trained and untrained males and females.

of aerobic training on the malate-aspartate and glycero-phosphate shuttle enzymes they also monitored CS activity in the quadriceps femoris muscle of the endurance-trained and untrained subjects. CS activity was 14.0 ± 1.4 mmol/min/kg after training compared to 8-9 $\pm$ 1.1 mmol/min/kg before training, an increase of 57%.

Again CS activity was shown to be elevated in human muscle following intense swim training in a 1989 study by Fitts, Costill, and Gardetto. Competitive swimmers trained 1.5 hours/day, 5 days/week, for 10 weeks, while participating in competition 1 day/week. Then at the end of the 10-week training period the training load was doubled for an additional 10 days, such that the men were training twice per day for 1.5 hours each session. Muscle biopsies from the posterior deltoid muscle were taken at 10 weeks and at 10 weeks plus 10 days. CS activity in a control group of sedentary subjects was 14.4 ± 0.3 mmol/min/kg compared to 26.2 ± 1.1 at 10 weeks of training and 28-6 $\pm$ 1.7 at 10 weeks plus 10 days ($p < 0.01$). This represented an 82% and 99% increase in CS activity for the trained and intensified trained muscles respectively.

Finally, mitochondrial CPK activity was elevated in the gastrocnemius muscle of both male and female marathon runners when compared to a group of nonrunning controls (Figure 8-11; Apple & Rogers, 1986). Thus, the enzyme adaptations occurring in human skeletal mus-

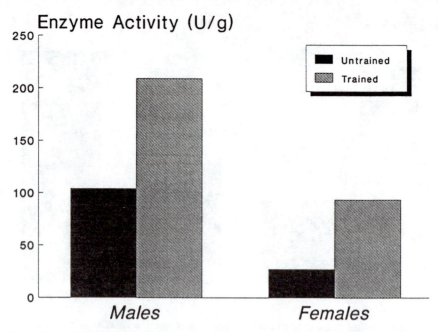

Figure 8-11. CPK activity in trained and untrained males and females.

cle following aerobic exercise training seem to be of the same type and magnitude as those seen following aerobic training in animals. In general, the key enzymes associated with the citric acid cycle, the electron transport chain, and fat oxidation increase about 100% with chronic aerobic training.

SUBSTRATE OXIDATION AFTER AEROBIC TRAINING

All of the enzymatic adaptations to aerobic training discussed above point to an increased ability for the muscle to produce ATP aerobically. Indeed, Yakovlev (1975) reported that prolonged endurance training increased the muscle's capacity to produce ATP by 30% when ATP production was expressed relative to mitochondrial protein, and by 85% when expressed relative to muscle protein. Although some investigators have shown a small increase (18 to 26%) in resting ATP concentration in trained muscle (Karlsson et al., 1972), this small increase in available ATP probably does not make a significant contribution to the energy supply needed during prolonged exercise. The real key to sustained energy production during prolonged exercise is the muscle's ability to oxidize carbohydrate and fat at a level equivalent to the energy demand during the exercise.

Holloszy (1967) was the first to compare values for oxygen con-

112   *BIOCHEMISTRY OF EXERCISE*

sumption between exercise-trained and untrained muscle. Using pyruvate + malate as a substrate, the mitochondrial fraction of trained gastrocnemius muscle consumed oxygen at a rate of 1022 ± 118 ml/hr/kg compared to 506 ± 53 ml/hr/kg for untrained muscle. The fact that the respiratory control index and the P:O ratios were similar between groups indicates that the increased capacity to consume oxygen was directly related to an ATP production.

Barnard, Edgerton, & Peter (1970) took the investigations a bit further and found that oxidative phosphorylation at the 3 sites within the electron transport chain was higher in trained muscle than untrained muscle. Guinea pigs were treadmill trained for 18 weeks, after which gastrocnemius and plantaris muscles were removed. Pyruvate + malate oxidation was increased by 65% in the trained muscle compared to untrained. When succinate + rotenone were incubated, oxygen consumption was elevated by 50% in the trained muscle. (Rotenone prevents ATP synthesis at site #1 by inhibiting electron transfer from NADH dehydrogenase to CoQ. Therefore synthesis of ATP can only occur at sites #2 and #3.) Oxidation of ascorbate was 61% higher in the trained muscle than in the untrained. (Ascorbate directly reduces cytochrome C, which effectively bypasses ATP synthesis sites #1 and #2.) The P:O ratio as well as the respiratory control index were similar between groups at all three ATP synthesis sites. This agrees with Holloszy's results (1967) in that training-induced elevations in oxygen consumption are accompanied by increased capacity for ATP production.

The focus of attention now turns to some specific substrates to see whether this increased oxidative capacity is general or substrate-specific. Molé and Holloszy (1970) were the first to show an increased capacity for fat oxidation following aerobic training. The gastrocnemius muscle from treadmill-trained rats exhibited an approximately 70% increase in palmitate oxidation over that of sedentary rats. A year later (1971), Molé, with Oscai and Holloszy, published another paper where they demonstrated that palmitate, oleate, linoleate, palmityl CoA, and palmityl carnitine oxidation capacities were increased with aerobic exercise training in both whole homogenates and the mitochondrial fractions of rat skeletal muscle (Figure 8-12).

Baldwin et al. (1972) made a significant contribution by showing that the capacity to oxidize carbohydrates (pyruvate) and lipids (palmitate) increased in three muscle types following aerobic training (Figure 8-13). Baldwin et al. (1975) again showed increases in pyruvate oxidation capacity following aerobic training. This time, however, the training stimulus was swimming. Rats were swim-trained for 6 hours/day, 5 days/week, for 14 weeks. Pyruvate oxidation rate in the exercised gastrocnemius muscle was only 35% greater than in the unexer-

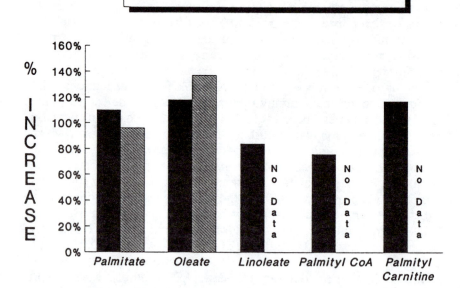

Figure 8-12. Capacity for fat oxidation in aerobically trained vs. untrained muscle.

cised muscle. This is quite a bit lower than the 116 to 157% increase seen with treadmill running (Figure 8-13). However, in another study, cell respiratory capacity following swim training was elevated by about 80% (Yakovlev, 1975), which is similar to what Holloszy (1967) reported for treadmill-trained rats. The Soviets have also seen great changes in the capacity to oxidize pyruvate (200%) and palmitate (120%), in addition to a 40% increase in succinate oxidation rate following prolonged exercise training (Yakovlev, 1975).

As mentioned earlier, ketone oxidation enzymes increase their activity in response to aerobic training (Winder, Baldwin, & Holloszy, 1975). This increase in enzyme activity is accompanied by an augmented rate of oxidation of 3-hydroxybutyrate (140%) and acetoacetate (90%). Clearly, the adaptations to aerobic exercise training in skeletal muscle are not specific to either lipid or carbohydrate oxidation but are general for all aerobic energy production.

SUBSTRATE STORAGE AFTER AEROBIC TRAINING

It seems logical that the substrate availability to the contracting muscle can play a critical role in energy production during prolonged exercise. Various studies have shown that resting glycogen stores are augmented in endurance-trained muscle (Figure 8-14; Gollnick et al., 1972;

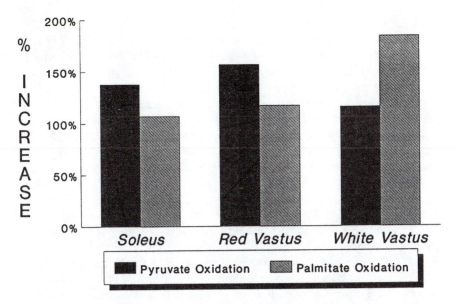

Figure 8-13. Capacity for pyruvate and palmitate oxidation in aerobically trained vs. untrained muscle.

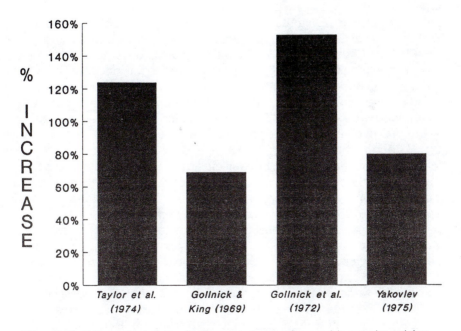

Figure 8-14. Enhancement of muscle glycogen storage after aerobic exercise training.

Gollnick & King, 1969; Taylor, Thayer, & Rao, 1972; Yakovlev, 1975). This increase in muscle glycogen storage following aerobic training is directly related to aerobic energy production per se and not to anaerobic glycolysis because maximal glycolytic rate is not elevated in aerobically trained muscle (Yakovlev, 1975). Furthermore, lactate levels in the muscle and blood are reduced during submaximal exercise following aerobic training (Baldwin et al., 1975; Karlsson et al., 1972). The mechanism behind the increased muscle glycogen storage following endurance training is a twofold increase in glycogen synthetase activity (Jefress, Peter, & Lamb, 1968; Taylor, Thayer, & Rao, 1972) as well as in glycogen branching enzyme activity (Taylor et al., 1974).

Depleted fat supply to the working muscle is not considered a factor in causing fatigue because of the abundant fat reserve found in the adipocytes. However, Morgan, Short and Cobb (1969) reported that long-term exercise caused an 83% increase in muscle triglyceride (TG) storage. These results are questionable because the training protocol used in this study was isotonic weight training, which isn't considered aerobic in nature. In contrast, Oscai, Caruso, and Wergeles (1982) reported that intracellular TG stores are reduced with training whereas intracellular free fatty acid content is elevated. Adding further to the confusion is the finding that glycerol 3-phosphate esterification into glycerides was increased in muscle of endurance-trained rats (Askew, Huston, & Dohm, 1973). One possible solution to this paradox is the idea that intramuscular TG stores are dynamic. It has been suggested that the intracellular TG storage pool within muscle is continually being turned over (Oscai et al., 1988). This means that, in order to determine the contribution of muscular TG to energy production, one must know the rate of TG turnover within the intracellular pool as well as the fate of all fatty acids entering the muscle cell. Until these parameters can be determined, we will not have a clear understanding of the role of intracellular TG in energy production during aerobic exercise.

Although all of the mechanisms behind the biochemical adaptations to aerobic training have not been elucidated, the substrate changes during submaximal exercise and their relationship to the enzymes important for lipid and carbohydrate metabolism have been described (Evans et al., 1979). Metabolic comparisons were made between a group of untrained males and a group of endurance-trained athletes (half of whom were competitive cyclists and half distance runners). Each subject was exercised for 60 minutes at a workload of 50% his respective $\dot{V}O_2$ max. Blood sampling revealed that circulating fatty acids increased to about the same extent in both groups, but that serum glycerol content was 125% higher in the trained athletes compared to controls. Serum TG, on the other hand, rose to a greater extent in the untrained men (24 mg%) than in the athletes (11 mg%). This blood lipid profile suggests that fatty acid turnover was greater in the trained men (evidenced by the elevated glycerol levels) and that the inability of the untrained men to utilize the fatty acids caused their reesterification into TG (evidenced by elevated serum TG).

Serum glucose was reduced by 5 mg% in the untrained men as compared to a rise of 11 mg% in the trained men. Muscle glycogen utilization was 23 mmoles for the trained, which was 44% less than the 34 mmoles used by the untrained. These findings along with others indicate that the enzymatic and substrate changes occurring in skeletal muscle in response to aerobic training produce a shift from carbohydrate to fat as the primary energy source for oxidative metabolism during submaximal exercise.

CONCLUSIONS

Figure 8-15 was created to help summarize the wealth of information relative to the biochemical adaptations occurring in skeletal muscle in response to aerobic training. Each panel of the figure represents a specific area of adaptation. Panel A deals with the adaptations in or relative to the electron transport chain. Panel B represents enzymatic adaptations relative to the citric acid cycle. Panel C shows enzyme changes specific to fat oxidation. Panel D presents data concerning oxidative capacity for specific substrates. The number in parentheses below each bar indicates the number of studies or groups from which the data was derived. In order to simplify the data, values were averaged across species, muscles, fiber types, and studies.

The following conclusions can be made about the biochemical adaptations in muscle following prolonged endurance training of an aerobic nature.

1. Components of the electron transport chain increase their capacity to produce ATP by about 100% following aerobic training.
2. Citric acid cycle related enzymes increase their activity to varying degrees (35 to 100$^+$%) following aerobic training.
3. Enzymes specific to fatty acid metabolism increase their activity by approximately 100% following aerobic training.
4. Ketone body enzymes also respond with about a 100% increase to aerobic training.
5. Mitochondrial CPK activity *may* increase up to twofold following aerobic training.
6. Enzymes of the malate-aspartate shuttle respond to aerobic training by increasing their activity, whereas the glycero-phosphate shuttle does not respond to training.

a. Electron Transport Markers

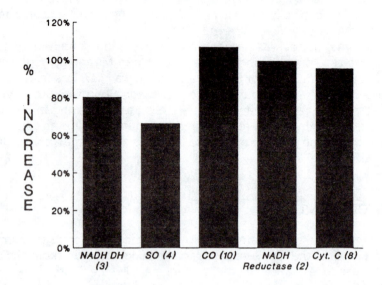

b. Citric Acid Cycle Related Enzymes

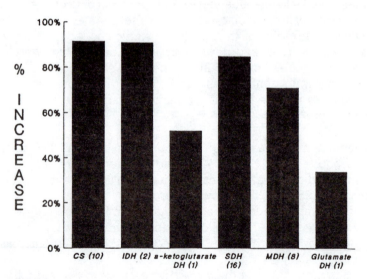

Figure 8-15. Biochemical adaptations in skeletal muscle following aerobic training.

c. Fatty Acid-Specific Enzymes

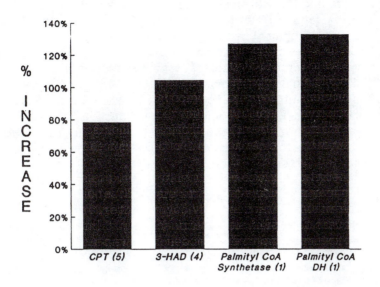

d. Substrate Oxidation Capacity

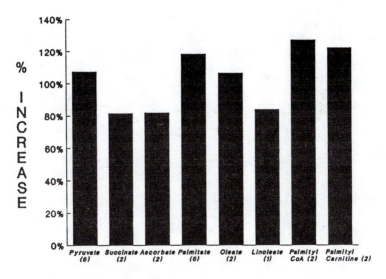

Figure 8-15 (continued)

7. Additional enzymes that respond to aerobic training are GPT, ATPase, and PK, with an increase in F1 ability to produce ATP.
8. The adaptations to aerobic training may be related to muscle fiber types or recruitment patterns during the exercise.
9. Increased capacity for aerobic metabolism is not substrate-specific.
10. Glycogen storage in aerobically trained muscle is 100 to 150% higher than in untrained muscle.
11. The overall aerobic training response in skeletal muscle is an increased capacity for aerobic energy production. Trained muscle exercising at submaximal workloads preferentially uses fat over carbohydrate to sustain the exercise, resulting in enhanced endurance exercise performance.

REFERENCES

Apple, F.S., & Rogers, M.A. (1986). Mitochondrial creatine kinase activity alterations in skeletal muscle during long-distance running. *J. Appl. Physiol.*, 61(2): 482-485.

Askew, E.W., Huston, R.L., & Dohm, G.L. (1973). Effect of physical training on esterification of glycerol-3-phosphate by homogenates of liver, skeletal muscle, heart, and adipose tissue of rats. *Metabolism*, 22(3): 473-480.

Baldwin, K.M., Fitts, R.H., Booth, F.W., Winder, W.W., & Holloszy, J.O. (1975). Depletion of muscle and liver glycogen during exercise: Protective effect of training. *Pflugers Arch.*, 354: 203-212.

Baldwin, K.M., Klinkerfuss, G.H., Terjung, R.L., & Molé, P.A. (1972). Respiratory capacity of white, red, and intermediate muscle: adaptative response to exercise. *Am. J. Physiol.*, 222(2): 373-378.

Baldwin, K.M., Winder, W.W., Terjung, R.L., & Holloszy, J.O. (1973). Glycolytic enzymes in different types of skeletal muscle: adaptation to exercise. *Am. J. Physiol.*, 225(4): 962-966.

Barnard, R.J., Edgerton, V.R., & Peter, J.B. (1970). Effect of exercise on skeletal muscle: I. Biochemical and histochemical properties. *J. Appl. Physiol.*, 28(6): 762-766.

Bertocci, L.A. & Gollnick, P.D. (1985). pH effect on mitochondria and individual enzyme function. *Med. Sci. Sports Exerc.*, 17(2): 244 (abstract).

Brooks, G.A. (1988). Blood lactic acid: sports "bad boy" turns good. *Gatorade Sports Science Exchange*, 1(2): 1-4.

Davies, K.J.A., Packer, L., & Brooks, G.A. (1981). Biochemical adaptation of mitochondria, muscle, and whole-animal respiration to endurance training. *Arch. Biochem. Biophys.*, 209(2): 539-554.

Evans, W.J., Bennett, A.S., Costill, D.L., & Fink, W.J. (1979). Leg muscle metabolism in trained and untrained men. *Res. Quart.*, 50(3): 350-359.

Fitts, R.H., Costill, D.L., & Gardetto, P.R. (1989). Effect of swim exercise training on human muscle fiber function. *J. Appl. Physiol.*, 66(1): 465-475.

Fournier, M., Ricci, J., Taylor, A.W., Ferguson, R.J., Montpetit, R.R., & Chaitman, B.R. (1982). Skeletal muscle adaptation in adolescent boys: sprint and endurance training and detraining. *Med. Sci. Sports Exerc.*, 14(6): 453-456.

Gollnick, P.D., Armstrong, R.B., Saltin, B., Saubert, C.W., IV, Sembrowich, W.L., & Shepherd, R.E. (1973). Effect of training on enzyme activity and fiber composition of human skeletal muscle. *J. Appl. Physiol.*, 34(1): 107-111.

Gollnick, P.D., Armstrong, R.B., Saubert, C.W., IV, Piehl, K., & Saltin, B. (1972). Enzyme activity and fiber composition in skeletal muscle of untrained and trained men. *J. Appl. Physiol.*, 33(3): 312-319.

Gollnick, P.D., & King, D.W. (1969). Effect of exercise and training on mitochondria of rat skeletal muscle. *Am. J. Physiol.*, 216(6): 1502-1509.

Green, H.J., Reichmann, H., & Pette, D. (1983). Fibre type specific transformations in the enzyme activity pattern of rat vastus lateralis muscle by prolonged endurance training. *Pflugers Arch.*, 399: 216-222.

Holloszy, J.O. (1967). Biochemical adaptations in muscle: Effects of exercise on mitochondrial oxygen uptake and respiratory enzyme activity in skeletal muscle. *J. Biol. Chem.*, 242(9): 2278-2282.

Holloszy, J.O. (1975). Adaptation of skeletal muscle to endurance exercise. *Med. Sci. Sports*, 7(3): 155-164.

Holloszy, J.O. & Oscai, L.B. (1969). Effect of exercise on α-glycerophosphate dehydrogenase activity in skeletal muscle. *Arch. Biochem. Biophys.*, 130: 653-656.

Holloszy, J.O., Oscai, L.B., Don, I.J., & Molé, P.A. (1970). Mitochondrial citric acid cycle and related enzymes: adaptive response to exercise. *Biochem. Biophys. Res. Comm.*, 40(6): 1368-1373.

Jefress, R.N., Peter, J.B., & Lamb, D.R. (1968). Effects of exercise on glycogen synthetase in red and white skeletal muscle. *Life Sci.*, 7(2): 957-960.

Karlsson, J., Nordesjo, L., Jorfeldt, L., & Saltin, B. (1972). Muscle lactate, ATP, and CP levels during exercise after physical training in man. *J. Appl. Physiol.*, 33(2): 199-203.

Mainwood, G.W. & Renaud, J.M. (1985). The effect of acid-base on fatigue of skeletal muscle. *Can. J. Physiol. Pharmacol.*, 63: 403-416.

Molé, P.A., Baldwin, K.M., Terjung, R.M., & Holloszy, J.O. (1973). Enzymatic pathways of pyruvate metabolism in skeletal muscle: adaptations to exercise. *Am. J. Physiol.*, 224(1): 50-54.

Molé, P.A. & Holloszy, J.O. (1970). Exercise-induced increase in the capacity of skeletal muscle to oxidize palmitate. *Pro. Soc. Exptl. Biol. Med.*, 134: 789-792.

Molé, P.A., Oscai, L.B., & Holloszy, J.O. (1971). Adaptation of muscle to exercise: Increase in levels of palmityl CoA syhthetase, carnitine palmityltransferase, and palmityl CoA dehydrogenase, and in the capacity to oxidize fatty acids. *J. Clin. Invest.*, 50: 2323-2330.

Morgan, T.E., Short, F.A., & Cobb, L.A. (1969). Effect of long-term exercise on skeletal muscle lipid composition. *Am. J. Physiol.*, 216(1): 82-86.

Orlander, J., Kiessling, J.-H., Karlsson, J., & Ekbolm, B. (1977). Low intensity training, inactivity, and resumed training in sedentary men. *Acta Physiol. Scand.*, 101: 351-362.

Oscai, L.B., Caruso, R.A., & Wergeles, A.C. (1982). Lipoprotein lipase hydrolyzes endogenous triacylglycerols in muscle of exercised rats. *J. Appl. Physiol.*, 52(4): 1059-1063.

Oscai, L.B., Gorski, J., Miller, W.C., & Palmer, W.K. (1988). Role of the alkaline TG lipase in regulating intramuscular TG content. *Med. Sci. Sports Exerc.*, 20(6): 539-544.

Oscai, L.B. & Holloszy, J.O. (1971). Biochemical adaptations in muscle: II Response of mitochondrial adenosine triphosphatase, creatine phosphokinase, and adenylate kinase activities in skeletal muscle to exercise. *J. Biol. Chem.*, 246(22): 6968-6972.

Oscai. L.B., Molé, P.A., Brei, B., & Holloszy, J.O. (1971). Cardiac growth and respiratory enzyme levels in male rats subjected to a running program. *Am. J. Physiol.*, 220(5): 1238-1241.

Schantz, P.G., Sjoberg, B., & Svedenhag, J. (1986). Malate-aspartate and alpha-glycerophosphate shuttle enzyme levels in human skeletal muscle: methodological considerations and effect of endurance training. *Acta Physiol. Scand.*, 128: 397-407.

Takekura, H. & Yoshioka, T. (1990). Different metabolic responses to exercise training programmes in single rat muscle fibres. *J. Muscle Res. Cell Motil.*, 11: 105-113.

Taylor, A.W., Stothart, J., Booth, M.A., Thayer, R., & Rao, S. (1974). Human skeletal muscle glycogen branching enzyme activities with exercise and training. *Can. J. Physiol. Pharmacol.*, 52: 119-122.

Taylor, A.W., Thayer, R., & Rao, S. (1972). Human skeletal muscle glycogen synthetase activities with exercise and training. *Can. J. Physiol. Pharmacol.*, 50: 411-415.

Winder, W.W., Baldwin, K.M., & Holloszy, J.O. (1974). Enzymes involved in ketone utilization in different types of muscle: adaptation to exercise. *Eur. J. Biochem.*, 47: 461-467.

Winder, W.W., Baldwin, K.M., & Holloszy, J.O. (1975). Exercise-induced increase in the capacity of rat skeletal muscle to oxidize ketones. *Can. J. Physiol. Pharmacol.*, 53: 86-91.

Yakovlev, N.N. (1975). Biochemistry of sport in the Soviet Union: beginning, development, and present status. *Med. Sci. Sports*, 7(4): 237-247.

Young, J.C. & Holloszy, J.O. (1983). Maintenance of the adaptation of skeletal muscle mitochondria to exercise in old rats. *Med. Sci. Sports Exerc.*, 15(3): 243-246.

9

ADAPTATIONS IN HORMONE RESPONSES FOLLOWING TRAINING

In Chapter 4 we briefly discussed the mechanisms by which epinephrine, norepinephrine, insulin, glucagon, and cortisol regulate energy production during muscular work. This hormonal regulation of exercise energy production represents a "whole body" response to muscular activity. Data presented in Chapters 5 through 8 represented the intramuscular adaptations to chronic exercise training. The increase in intramuscular resources for energy production following training reduces the necessity for the activation of a whole body response to submaximal exercise. This suggests that the hormonal response to submaximal exercise may be eliminated or greatly reduced following exercise training.

An example of this reduced hormonal response following training has been demonstrated for the catecholamines by Winder et al. (1978). Six male subjects trained aerobically for 7 weeks by cycling and/or running 30 to 50 minutes/day. Prior to training and after training the participants were subjected to a 5-minute bicycle ergometer test at about 95% of their pre-training $\dot{V}O_2$ max. Figure 9-1 illustrates how the normal exercise-induced rise in circulating catecholamines was diminished following training. This adaptation in hormonal response to exercise was manifest as early as 1 week into the training period and leveled off after about 3 weeks.

A year later the same investigators demonstrated that this diminished hormonal response to exercise at the same absolute workload following training was also apparent for relative workloads (Winder et al., 1979). Six male subjects trained aerobically for 9 weeks as in the previous study (Winder et al., 1978). Pre- and post-training blood samples were taken immediately after a 90-minute exercise bout at an intensity of $58 \pm 2\%$ of initial $\dot{V}O_2$ max as well as at $62 \pm 2\%$ of final $\dot{V}O_2$ max. Figure 9-2 shows that at the same absolute workload the hormonal response to the exercise bout was reduced following training. This blunted hormonal response to exercise after training was also

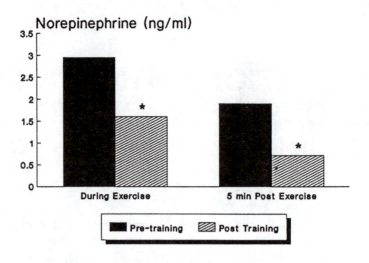

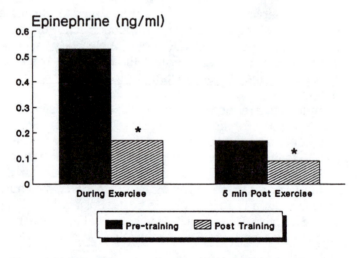

Figure 9-1. Catecholamine response to exercise following aerobic training. *Significantly different from pre-training, $p < 0.05$.

manifest at similar relative workloads for epinephrine and glucagon, but not for norepinephrine.

Other researchers have also found that sympathetic nervous activity (plasma norepinephrine concentration) during exercise remains constant in relation to relative workload, but is reduced in reference to absolute workload following training (Peronnet et al., 1981). Ten sedentary males trained for 20 weeks on a bicycle ergometer 3 days/week, for 30 minutes/day, at a workload of 80% maximal heart rate. Plasma

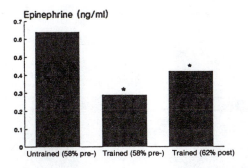

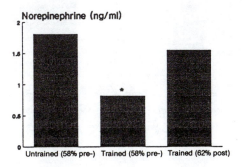

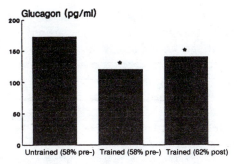

Figure 9-2. Hormonal response to absolute and relative exercise workloads following aerobic training.

*Significantly different from untrained, p<0.05.

norepinephrine levels were 50% lower post-training when the samples were taken at similar absolute workloads. However, at similar relative workloads, norepinephrine levels pre- and post-training were equivalent (Figure 9-3).

Reduced epinephrine levels were seen in blood samples of competitive swimmers following 9 weeks of training when determined at similar relative workloads of high intensity (200 yard swim at maximal

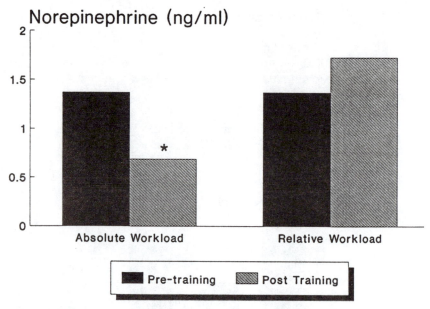

Figure 9-3. Norepinephrine response to absolute and relative exercise workloads following aerobic training.
    *Significantly different from pre-training, $p < 0.05$.

effort) as well as when determined at similar absolute workloads of moderate intensity (1,000 yard swim at the same pace pre- and post-training). However, these scientists saw no training effect upon plasma norepinephrine concentrations (Hickson et al., 1979).

Glucagon is a pancreatic hormone that increases the rate of glycogenolysis. During prolonged exercise when blood glucose levels may be compromised, glucagon levels will increase to aid in the maintenance of blood glucose. One might expect that as the cellular adaptations to prolonged exercise training favor reduced glucose-derived energy production during exercise, that the glucagon response to acute exercise would be blunted following a period of aerobic training. Indeed, this has been the case when untrained individuals undertake a vigorous training program (Figure 9-2; Winder et al., 1979). However, competitive swimmers who undertook 9 weeks of training showed no training adaptation in their glucagon response to a single exercise bout (Hickson et al., 1979).

Insulin, which is a glucagon antagonist, increases fat and glycogen storage and lowers blood glucose levels; these actions are counter-productive during exercise. Therefore, as one may expect, the dramatic drop in blood insulin levels seen during exercise in untrained individuals is attenuated with training. For example, plasma insulin levels of exercise-trained men were 56% higher following training than prior to training when measured at a given absolute workload (Winder et al., 1979).

The mechanism behind this reduced insulin response to a single exercise bout following training is most likely an increased insulin sensitivity produced by training (Dolkas, Rodnick, & Mondon, 1990; Farrell, 1988; Mikines et al., 1987). This was just recently demonstrated by Farrell (1988). Rats were trained to run on a treadmill 5 days/week at 32 meters/minute for 90 minutes. Following 8 weeks of training, hyperglycemic glucose clamps at 11 mM for 90 min resulted in elevations in plasma insulin to 23.6 ± 4.3 ng/ml for sedentary rats compared to 11.8 ± 1.1 ng/ml for the trained rats. This increased sensitivity to insulin persists for at least 7 days after cessation of exercise training (Dolkas, Rodnick, & Mondon, 1990).

The effect of exercise training on cortisol release during exercise is not clear. Much of the research points in the direction of a reduced response in cortisol release following training (Shephard & Sidney, 1975). However, others have shown an increased response following training (Fellmann et al., 1985).

CONCLUSIONS

During a single bout of exercise the hormones that increase the rate of lipolysis, glycogenolysis, and gluconeogenesis will be elevated, whereas those that increase energy storage tend to be decreased. The magnitude of changes in these hormonal alterations is not as great after training as before training. This "blunted" hormonal response during exercise after training appears to be related more to the absolute workload than the relative workload. In consequence, the threshold intensity for activation of hormonal response is elevated following training. The mechanism behind these adaptations could be alterations in hormone metabolism and/or altered sensitivity to the hormones by the target tissue.

[A complete review of the hormonal adaptations to exercise training is beyond the focus and scope of this book. For an in depth review the reader is referred to the work of Viru (1985)].

REFERENCES

Dolkas, C.B., Rodnick, K.J., & Mondon, C.E. (1990). Effect of body weight gain on insulin sensitivity after retirement from exercise training. *J. Appl. Physiol.*, 68(2): 520-526.

Farrell, P.A. (1988). Decreased insulin response to sustained hyperglycemia in exercise-trained rats. *Med. Sci. Sports Exerc.*, 20(5): 469-473.

Fellmann, N., Coudert, J., Jarrige, J.-F., Bedu, M., Denis, C., Boucher, D., & Lacour, J.-R. (1985). Effects of endurance training on the androgenic response to exercise in man. *Int. J. Sports Med.*, 6(4): 215-219.

Hickson, R.C., Hagberg, J.M., Conlee, R.K., Jones, D.A., Ehsani, A.A., & Winder, W.W. (1979). Effect of training on hormonal responses to exercise in competitive swimmers. *Eur. J. Appl. Physiol.*, 41: 211-219.

Mikines, K.J., Dela, F., Sonne, B., Farrell, P.A., Richter, E.A., & Galbo, H. (1987). Insulin action and secretion in man: effects of different levels of physical activity. *Can. J. Spt. Sci.*, 12(Suppl. 1): 113S-116S.

Peronnet, F., Cleroux, J., Perrault, H., Cousineau, D., de Champlain, J., & Nadeau, R. (1981). Plasma norepinephrine response to exercise before and after training in humans. *J. Appl. Physiol.*, 51(4): 812-815.

Shephard, R.J. & Sidney, K.H. (1975). Effects of exercise on plasma growth hormone and cortisol levels in human subjects. In J.H. Wilmore (ed.), *Exercise and Sports Sciences Reviews: Vol. 3*, pp. 1-31. New York; Academic Press.

Viru, A. (1985). *Hormones in muscular activity: Volume 2, Adaptive effect of hormones in exercise*. Boca Raton, FL: CRC Press.

Winder, W.W., Hagberg, J.M., Hickson, R.C., Ehsani, A.A., & McLane, J.A. (1978). Time course of sympathoadrenal adaptation to endurance exercise training in man. *J. Appl. Physiol.*, 45(3): 370-374.

Winder, W.W., Hickson, R.C., Hagberg, J.M., Ehsani, A.A., & McLane, J.A. (1979). Training-induced changes in hormonal and metabolic responses to submaximal exercise. *J. Appl. Physiol.*, 46(4): 766-771.

Appendix A:

Common Biochemical Abbreviations

ACP	acyl carrier protein
ADP	adenosine diphosphate
AK	adenylate kinase
AMP	adenosine monophosphate
AT	aspartate transaminase
ATP	adenosine triphosphate
ATPase	adenosine triphosphatase
cAMP	cyclic AMP
CAP	carnitine acyl transferase
CO	cytochrome oxidase
CoA	coenzyme A
COOH	carboxyl group of an amino acid
CoQ	coenzyme Q
CPK	creatine phosphokinase
CPT	carnitine palmityltransferase
CS	citrate synthase
DHAP	dihydroxyacetone phosphate
DNA	deoxyribonucleic acid
FAD	flavin adenine dinucleotide (oxidized form)
$FADH_2$	flavin adenine dinucleotide (reduced form)
FMN	flavin mononucleotide
GPT	glutamate-pyruvate transaminase
GTP	guanosine triphosphate
3-HAD	3-hydroxyacyl coenzyme A dehydrogenase
HCO_3	bicarbonate
HK	hexokinase
HSL	hormone-sensitive lipase
IDH	isocitrate dehydrogenase
IP_3	D-myo-inositol 1,4,5-triphosphate
LDH	lactate dehydrogenase
LPL	lipoprotein lipase

129

MDH	malate dehydrogenase
MK	myokinase
NAD^+	nicotinamide adenine dinucleotide (oxidized form)
NADH	nicotinamide adenine dinucleotide (reduced form)
$NADP^+$	nicotinamide adenine dinucleotide phosphate (oxidized form)
NADPH	nicotinamide adenine dinucleotide phosphate (reduced form)
NH_2	amino radical of an amino acid
NH_4^+	ammonia
PC	phosphocreatine
PFK	phosphofructokinase
Pi	inorganic phosphate
PK	pyruvate kinase
SDH	succinate dehydrogenase
SO	succinate oxidase
TG	triacylglycerol or triglyceride
UDP	uridine diphosphate
UTP	uridine triphosphate

Appendix B:
Cross-Reference With Exercise Physiology Texts

The following table cross-references the chapters of this book with chapters in common exercise physiology books that this book can supplement.

Miller	A&R	B&F	deV	FBF	Lam	MKK	Nob	P&H	W&C
1. Skeletal Muscle	2, 3	19	2, 4, 5	5, 6	3	18, 19	1, 2	8	1, 5
2. Energy	7, 12	4-8	3	2	4	1, 5-7	3	3	2
3. Energy Storage	12	5, 7	—	3	4	—	4	—	8
4. Energy Regulation	7, 12	5-9	10	22	4, 17	6, 20	3	3, 4, 5	2, 6
5. Structural Adaptation	2, 10	6, 20	2	5	3	22	1, 14	8	1, 7, 8
6. ATP-PC Adaptation	7, 10, 12	4	3	13	4, 14	6, 21	14	3, 19	8
7. Glycolytic Adaptation	7, 10, 12	5	3	13	4, 14	6, 21	14	3, 19	8
8. Aerobic Adaptation	10, 12	5-8	3, 19	13	4, 10	6, 21	14	3, 13, 19	8
9. Hormone Adaptation	10, 12	9	10	22	17	20	3	5	6

A&R = Astrand, P.O., and Rodahl, K. (1986). *Textbook of Work Physiology Physiological Bases of Exercise* (3rd ed.). New York; McGraw-Hill.
B&F = Brooks, G.A. and Fahey, T.D. (1984). *Exercise Physiology Human Bioenergetics and Its Applications.* New York; Wiley.
deV = de Vries, H.A. (1986). *Physiology of Exercise* (4th ed.). Dubuque, IA; William C. Brown.
FBF = Fox, E.L, Bowers, R.W., & Foss, M.L. (1989). *The Physiological Basis of Physical Education and Athletics* (4th ed.). Dubuque, IA: Wm. C. Brown.
Lam = Lamb, D.R. (1984). *Physiology of Exercise Responses & Adaptations* (2nd ed.). New York; Macmillan.
MKK = McArdle, W.D, Katch, F.I., & Katch, V.L. (1991). *Exercise Physiology Energy, Nutrition, and Human Performance* (3rd ed.). Philadelphia; Lea & Febiger.
Nob = Noble, B.J. (1986). *Physiology of Exercise and Sport.* St. Louis, MO; Times Mirror/Mosby.
P&H = Powers, S.K. and Howley, E.T. (1990). *Exercise Physiology Theory and Application to Fitness and Performance.* Dubuque, IA; William C. Brown.
W&C = Wilmore, J.H, and Costill, D.L. (1988). *Training for Sport and Activity* (3rd ed.). Dubuque, IA; William C. Brown.

Index